Before They Ask

From the Editor

In a letter accompanying their submission of the final revision of this book, writers Don and Rhoda Preston noted the feeling that they now had *three* children—Kathryn, Timothy, and BEFORE THEY ASK. As an editor, I am impressed by the thorough research, the biblical understanding, the Christian warmth and humor, and the commitment to a positive attitude toward sexuality that Don and Rhoda bring to their writing. As a parent, I am challenged by their insights and reassured by their experiences.

Don, a former school teacher, music educator, and budget analyst, is a United Methodist pastor, currently serving in Dickinson, North Dakota. He plays slow pitch softball, directs a barbershop chorus, and enjoys canoeing. Rhoda is a free-lance writer and music teacher with an undergraduate degree in biology and chemistry, is active in the United Methodist Women, loves sewing and tennis, and does not enjoy canoeing. Both are graduates of Austin Presbyterian Theological Seminary. Eleven-year-old Kathryn and seven-year-old Timothy have willingly contributed their experiences to the pages that follow.

I join Don and Rhoda in the hope that you who read this book and who participate in study groups will find both affirmation and inspiration for the demanding task of parenting. God's blessings as you prepare to respond to the needs of your children and to answer their questions, BEFORE THEY ASK.

James H. Ritchie, Jr.
Editor, BEFORE THEY ASK

Rhoda Preston

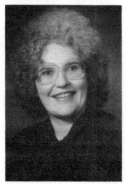

Don Preston

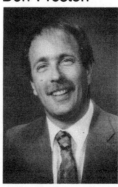

Before They Ask

TALKING ABOUT SEX
FROM A CHRISTIAN PERSPECTIVE

A Guide for Parents of Children
From Birth Through Age Twelve

Written by Don and Rhoda Preston

Illustrated by Dennis Jones

Contents

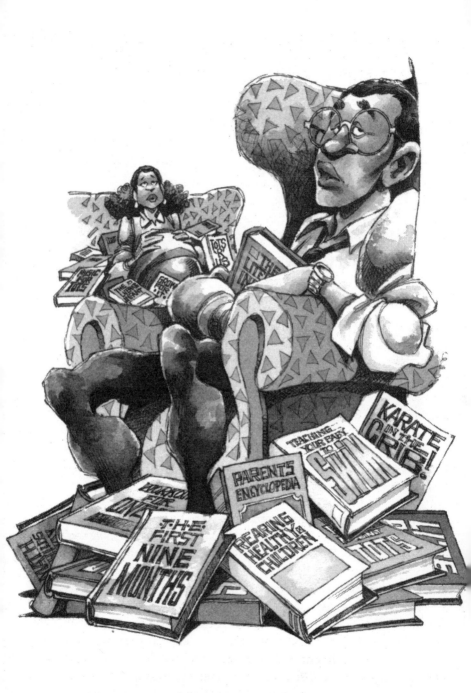

"Next on the list: Sex Education!"

CHAPTER 1

HOPES AND EXPECTATIONS

Expectant Parents

One October afternoon twelve years ago, our doctor leaned across his desk, reached over pictures of his own five children, grabbed our hands, started shaking them enthusiastically, and with a voice and a smile as bright as his blue golfing pants, spoke the words we had hoped for: "Congratulations, Don and Rhoda! You're expectant parents!" His good news left us feeling dizzy with anticipation and joy.

We were exuberant with expectations! What great hopes and dreams we had for this yet-to-be-born child! *Our* baby, of course, would be happy, healthy, and wholly cherished—we would be intentional about that. With a band director for a father and a mother who taught piano and organ, our little girl or boy was automatically expected to be musical. We also expected that this new family member would enjoy sports, devour books, love God, and make friends easily. We pledged that our son or daughter would be raised in a home that was free from sexual stereotypes. We bought colorful, stimulating toys for the nursery and read every book we could find on parenting—expecting that our efforts would result in a child who was exceptionally perceptive and alert.

Though our children, Kathryn and Timothy, are now eleven and seven, we are *still* expectant parents! We expect so much of our son and daughter. We hope they will each have a strong self-image and every chance for fulfillment. We want them to form positive relationships and to develop the capacity to give and to receive love. We are eager that they learn to think and that they become persons of integrity and kindness. We also expect a lot of ourselves as parents. We expect that we will be able to communicate our Christian values with our children. We expect that we will encourage the fulfillment of their dreams and will learn and grow from their insights. And *still* we find ourselves pouring over books on parenting, always expecting that one day we'll know how it's done.

Expectations and Concerns About Our Child's Gender

Before Kathryn's birth, friends would ask, "What are you hoping for—a boy or a girl?" While we would answer, "Oh, it doesn't matter. As long as it's healthy," Rhoda secretly hoped for a girl. The idea of raising a boy frightened her. How did little boys think and feel? She wasn't sure. She had a wonderful brother, but since he was six years older, she had not known him as a little boy.

A baby girl would be different—something far less mysterious. "After all," Rhoda thought, "I was once a little girl. My best childhood friends were my sisters. I'm close to my own mother. I'm comfortable with being female." Raising a male child would be a journey into strange and even frightening new territory!

Concerns about the gender of an unborn child are common. Gender—being male or female—tends to lock us into roles that are largely determined by the expectations of the society in which we live. Society assigns a set of rights, duties, and appropriate behaviors to males and females and thus defines for each a separate role in that culture. How a person then feels about himself or herself is influenced by those standards.

The assignment of these separate sets of rights, duties, and appropriate behaviors has caused parents to prefer having children of one sex instead of the other. For example, since the time recorded in the Hebrew Bible, many families have desired a son to carry on the family name. A familiar story from the fifteenth chapter of Genesis deals with Abram's longing for a son. When God promised Abram a great reward for his faithfulness, Abram told God in no uncertain terms that God's reward would mean nothing without a son to inherit that reward.

Parents may have other reasons for preferring a child of a particular gender. For example, a woman who has been denied opportunities because of her gender may prefer to have a son, anticipating that a daughter would be forced to contend with similar career or educational limitations. Likewise, a man who has been constantly pressured by his father and grandfather to excel in sports or in the family business may fear that such pressures will be passed on to his son. He may personally wish for a daughter, hoping to break the chain of pressure.

In the United States, gender preference may be of a more practical nature. Parents may find it easier or less expensive to have a child of a certain sex. For example, following the birth of her third son, one of our friends was visited by a well-intentioned neighbor who came to extend sympathy. The neighbor was convinced that Jane would be devastated by the tragedy of not having at least one daughter. "Actually," Jane said, "I was relieved. I'm a expert now on boys. And besides, we won't have to buy all new baby clothes."

Parents' Expectations About Their Child's Sexuality

Parents are not only concerned about their child's gender role, but also have expectations and hopes about their child's sexuality. Sexuality includes the physical and emotional aspects of being male or female. It is experienced in our hearts and minds as well as in our bodies. More than being simply the act of sexual intercourse, sexuality is an inclusive part of who we are as human beings. It informs our ethics, colors our desires, influences our actions, and defines our relationships.

A positive understanding and expression of sexuality is crucial for a life of fulfillment and joy. This is what loving parents want for their children. Parents wish to help their son or daughter to experience a life in which sexuality is a vibrant and healthy force. Knowing that problems with sexuality can cause pain and sorrow, wise parents strive to help their children avoid potential problems.

Such parents know it is unreasonable to assume that sexual understanding will come innately to their children. Appropriate meanings, values, actions, and feelings about sexuality must be learned. While Sunday school and church, schools, and peer groups all convey this information, the privilege of serving as the primary sex educators for children belongs to parents.

Parents as the Primary Sex Educators

What would it really mean for a parent to accept the responsibility for this sex education? Would it mean trying to control and suppress sexual expression to ensure that a child would always stay out of trouble? No, not primarily. Would it mean drilling children on the facts of life? sitting with infants and memorizing sex vocabulary flashcards: "These are the fallopian tubes. This is an ovary"? No, of course not. We are definitely not advocating all the "courses" suggested by the cartoon at the opening of this chapter! Bombarding young children with such learning activities is neither appropriate nor helpful. We do not recommend such an approach with any subject—including the subject of sexuality.

On the other hand, responsible parents do not postpone sex education, planning to schedule one quick crash course discussion about the birds and the bees at a point when they have determined that their child is old enough. Effective sex education involves building self-esteem and helping children understand and accept themselves as sexual beings. This approach calls for a lifetime view of a child's sexuality. It enables the child to say "No" to sexual contact today and an enthusiastic "Yes" to a full and mature expression of his or her sexuality in the future.

Responsible sex education would mean enabling your children to use their sexual knowledge in a responsible manner, making wise decisions and alleviating ignorance, misinformation, fear, and negative attitudes. It would mean providing an open, warm, and caring atmosphere so that children could see healthy relationships and appreciate the love and importance of the family.

According to The American Association of Sex Educators, Counselors and Therapists (AASEPT), there are several areas of basic concern which need to be included in sex education. One key area is information about human reproduction—including information about menstruation, conception, contraception, and pregnancy. Another area is the explanation of developmental changes that occur as a person grows—changes which might raise anxieties about whether or not one is normal.

Most professional sex educators appear to agree that children should have a solid understanding of these two areas (reproduction and the physical changes of puberty) before reaching junior high school. As adolescents, they are then free to focus on the development of relationships, attitudes, and values. The implication here is that most parents, churches, and schools wait far too long before beginning sex education. Then, to make matters worse, the instruction in sex education often ends with the acquisition of biological facts, without giving children the assistance they need to form their own values.

Living Day by Day

Our desire to provide positive sexuality training for our families leads us to examine the ways we relate to our children in other areas. Life cannot be compartmentalized. Each part of our lives is shaped and influenced by every other part. Our experiences intertwine to shape and form us as whole persons. A suggestion, then, for family sex education would be this: *Gain good general parenting skills.* The purpose of the remainder of this chapter is to suggest what some of those general parenting skills might be and to show how each may influence our child's sexual identity.

Helping Our Children to Know God

One of the privileges of Christian parenting is helping our children to know God personally. Do they know that God loves and values them? This assurance can be the foundation for a self-esteem that will enable them to love themselves. Have we helped our children discover what the Bible says about life and relationships? Its stories can guide actions and influence values. Do our sons and daughters know how to pray? Have they experienced the wisdom, peace, and power from time spent alone with God? Helping our children build a vital relationship with God means that we must talk with them about God and must also model a set of values based on our understanding of Christian love. We can make the Scriptures and prayer a natural part of our daily lives, using them as a source of wisdom and as instruction for self-control.

Family Atmosphere

One of the important ingredients in any home is family atmosphere. How does it feel to be present in your home? Do the members of your family experience security, gentleness, caring, and intimacy? Are family members "kind and tenderhearted to one another" (Ephesians 4:32a)? Do parents and children alike know what it means to be valued and loved? Does your family enjoy being together, so that members are comfortable and happy being part of the family? Do you experience occasional moments of joy together? Do you have a sense of family identity and pride?

Children who know from birth—or experience from conception—what it means to be cherished and loved are apt to grow into adults who accept God's love and extend this love to others. They will realize how important family loyalty is and will have had opportunity to practice building and sustaining joyful relationships. Such children will understand how to think in terms of *we* instead of *me* and will have had experience in demonstrating patience, flexibility, and concern for the well-being of others.

Listen to Philippians 2:1-4 and hear how Paul's words speak to the way in which Christian persons can develop a warm and loving atmosphere in their homes:

> Your life in Christ makes you strong, and his love comforts you. You have fellowship with the Spirit, and you have kindness and compassion for one another. I urge you, then, to make me completely happy by having the same thoughts, sharing the same love, and being one in soul and mind. Don't do anything from selfish ambition, or from a cheap desire to boast, but be humble toward one another, always considering others better than yourselves. And look out for one another's interests, not just for your own.

A Christian family who endeavors to exhibit the love of Christ in their home will be working to put this kindness, consideration, and loving unity into practice every day.

A warm family atmosphere can provide the basis for learning to handle emotions. Parents who say, "It looks to me like you're feeling sad (or discouraged, or excited, or angry, or afraid . . .)" are teaching their children to be sensitive to the feelings of others. Adults who attempt to figure out the source of emotions—especially those that accompany growing up—are teaching their children to be thoughtful and reasonable. Such children will, hopefully, be better prepared to react responsibly to their own feelings and will be at an advantage when it comes to handling the emotional aspects of a relationship.

The story of Nehemiah in the Bible is an example of how sensitivity to the feelings of others and the practice of emotional discipline can have a positive effect on a person's life. Nehemiah, the wine steward for Emperor Artaxerxes of Persia, was usually a happy person. Yet one day the emperor was surprised to see his servant looking sad. Nehemiah recounts the story with these words:

> (Artaxerxes) had never seen me look sad before, so
> he asked, "Why are you looking so sad? You
> aren't sick, so it must be that you're unhappy." I
> was startled. (Nehemiah 2:1-2).

Nehemiah was amazed that his feelings were noticed by the emperor. The emperor's sensitivity left Nehemiah free to answer "Yes, I am unhappy." He told Artaxerxes of his grief over the destruction of Jerusalem, and together they came up with a solution. The emperor gave Nehemiah the opportunity to change the circumstances that were causing his unhappiness, granting him permission to return to Jerusalem and oversee the rebuilding of the city. The insight and sensitivity of Artaxerxes and the willingness of Nehemiah to come to grips with his feelings give a positive model for parents and children to explore as they wrestle with their own feelings.

Building Self-Esteem

Families need to appreciate and value each member. Healthy self-esteem enables a person to develop and grow psychologically, laying a foundation for success in almost every area of life. Self-esteem contributes to feelings of competence, worth, and acceptance, and enhances the formation of meaningful relationships—relationships founded on mutual love and respect. Without self-esteem, it is difficult for persons to love themselves, to overcome fear of rejection or inferiority, or to accept their own limitations as well as the limitations of others. Children who have positive thoughts about themselves grow to become more positive adults! This is a gift we cannot afford to withhold from our children.

How can we build self-esteem in our daughters and sons? We can care for their physical needs. We can let them know through our explicit words and actions that they are cherished and respected. We can say, "let's do something together", showing our children that we value their company. We can find an hour in our busy schedule to volunteer for a school carnival, or to decorate two dozen cupcakes for a Valentine party. We can give our children the freedom to be unique and not insist that they be a carbon copy of their brothers and sisters or parents. We can ask for their assistance, for their ideas, and for their opinions. We can accept their differences of opinion without feeling angry or threatened. We can give our sons and daughters a voice in family decisions, celebrate their successes, and thank them for their help. We can tell them, "what you just did made me very happy, and I appreciate you greatly."

In our family, we often use memories to celebrate the uniqueness of each person. Kathy and Timothy like to look in their baby books to see the many cards of congratulation that were sent at their birth. We enjoy browsing through old photographs and saying: "Remember when you made your first soccer goal? Remember how much you loved your first kitten?" We try to make birthdays an especially happy time, and say "Remember the year we went to the professional baseball game on your birthday? Remember your 'Sleeping Beauty' cake?" We talk about special times we have shared and encourage our children to find ways to remember their experiences and feelings—through keeping diaries or having a dresser drawer for pictures and papers too precious to part with.

When we work at building our children's self-esteem, we are helping them to know that there is something special about them that no one else can duplicate. We are reinforcing their conviction that their bodies, as well as their entire selves, are good! We believe that this realization will help our children form mature attitudes about their sexuality and prepare them to make loving, lifetime commitments when they become adults!

Communication Skills

Throughout this book, we will be stressing the importance of family communication. We believe that children who feel comfortable talking with their parents about fears, fantasies, hopes, and frustrations will also be open to talking about sexuality. Families that have a history of listening to one another will continue to listen when the concerns are physical changes or sexual relationships. Families that communicate will find it easier to make decisions and resolve conflicts.

To communicate effectively, family members must first take time to be together. It is hard to have a relaxed conversation when no one has the time to listen. Set aside moments just to be together, to enjoy one another's company. Take the phone off the hook or plan an outing to the park. Driving in the car can provide a good opportunity to talk. Such settings have the potential for becoming some of your best opportunities for communication.

Many families find that it helps to be *doing* something together when you talk. Having a task eases self-consciousness and lessens tension, making it easier to talk. Working together also creates a feeling of support and rapport between family members—an important basis for open discussions. Just make sure you don't get so caught up in the project that you can't "bother" to talk!

Putting thoughts and feelings into words is often difficult; families must learn to be good listeners. Listening helps the words to come. Listening takes energy, alertness, and concentration. A good listener is interested and shows this interest with eye contact or a smile. A good listener pays attention to what is said and notes facial expressions and tone of voice which may give special meaning to the words. Listening gives us valuable information about one another. Listening also sends the message that the listener cares, and it makes the person who is talking feel important and accepted.

Parents often need to encourage their children to communicate. Parents can draw their child out by saying, "Susie, you look sad," or "Bryan, you must be very proud to have scored the winning goal!" Once children have started to open up, we can encourage them to keep talking by nodding, by saying, "I see" or "that's interesting— go on," or by occasionally asking an appropriate question.

Parents also need to make sure they are accurately hearing and interpreting what their child says. Do not assume that you understand. If you are not certain, ask about it. You might use your child's own words, but rephrase them in the form of a question. Or, you could comment on the implied content or feelings of the child's message:

Child: "I hate that stupid Richy. He makes me feel so dumb."

Parent: "It sounds as if he really hurt your feelings."

Responding in this way is similar to being a mirror. Your response reflects the attitudes or feelings that you hear, giving the child the chance to say, "Yes, that's it" or "No, what I mean is . . . ." Such responses encourage your children to continue to talk to you. It makes them feel that their feelings are respected and understood and helps them to identify the source of their emotions or problems.

There are some responses, frequently used by parents, that are basically conversation-stoppers. You may say, "Oh, just forget about it," or "Tomorrow's another day," or "You shouldn't feel that way," fully intending to help a child feel better. But such phrases often stop the conversation by denying the depth of the child's feelings. Children will feel as if their worries are unimportant and may decide that their parents don't understand or aren't interested.

Another type of conversation-stopper is to place blame and criticize. When parents respond to a child's conversation by saying, "That's ridiculous!" or "Wherever did you get *that* crazy idea?," the child will feel inferior and inadequate. This negative criticism hurts and is a strong incentive to keep things to yourself.

We parents don't always have to be on the listening end of a conversation. We can express our own thoughts, can put labels on our feelings, and can feel free to say, "I've got this problem. Maybe you can help me figure out a solution." We can say, "This is how I've always looked at this issue, but I may be wrong. What do you think?" By showing our children that we need someone to talk to, parents can demonstrate how important talking things out can be for adult relationships. It also gives our children the opportunity to practice good listening skills as they respond to us. This does not mean that we should burden young children with adult worries or expect them to have the wisdom and understanding that only maturity can bring. But we can be open, honest, and human, and gain from the insight and care of our children.

Perhaps the most important thing that parents can do is to remember that each child is a gift and a trust—not a possession. We are responsible for loving our children, for giving them our highest respect, and for making clear our values. But we do not own them. Our sons and daughters are entrusted to us. With the gift of children, God provides us with the opportunity to help shape and to be shaped by them. Instead of wanting to limit our children, we can give them some of the greatest gifts possible: the freedom to feel, to think, to inquire, and to choose.

The Story of Hannah

The story of Hannah found in 1 Samuel is an example of one mother who was able to be this kind of parent. Hannah longed for a child. She acknowledged to herself, to her husband, and even to Eli the priest that she felt empty, hurt, bitter, and sad. She spent time in prayer, telling God her dreams and her sorrows. When at last little Samuel was born, Hannah realized that this child was a gift from God. She was thrilled to have his life entrusted to her and did everything that modern authorities say a nurturing mother should do: she cuddled Samuel, held him close to nurse, surrounded him with her love. But Hannah knew that she had no right to own, keep, or limit her son. She knew that his relationship with God came first.

It must have been difficult for Hannah to take Samuel to live at the temple, but that is what she did. She carefully passed on to him the necessary skills to be self-assured and competent. She trusted his ability to think for himself. She taught him to be faithful to God and to care about right living. She took care of his physical needs, lovingly sewing his new clothes, then stepped back and let him go.

A Prayer of Hope and Expectation

Loving God, we come to you as expectant parents, filled with hopes and dreams for our children. We want them to be happy and fulfilled, to have strong self-images and a respect and appreciation for their bodies. We want them to know how to give and receive love.

Help us not to limit our children, but to be aware and supportive of their unique identity. Give us the wisdom and courage to pass on our Christian values—not just about sex, but about all of life. Help us to be loving in our families, enabling our children to discover and to experience the beauty of intimate relationships.

And most of all, like Hannah in the Old Testament, let us never forget that children are your gift and trust to us. Enable us to be faithful to our children and to you. Amen.

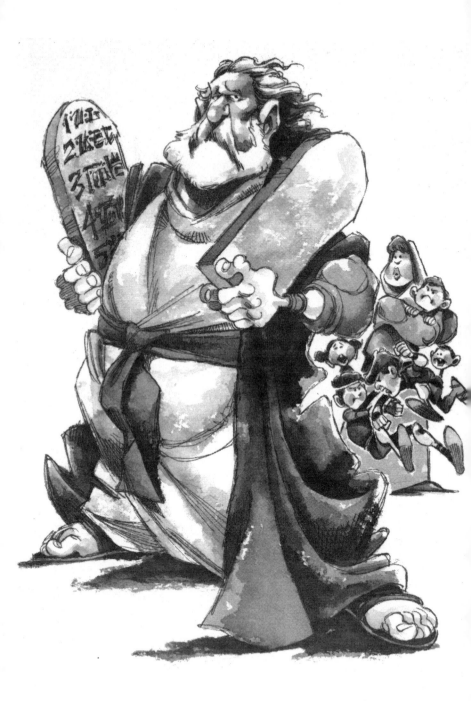

"Next time you're up there, how about getting
Ten Steps To Successful Parenting?"

CHAPTER 2

KNOWING, DECIDING AND BEING IN CONTROL

Decision-Making Skills

When Kathryn was two years old, our friend Mark was pushing her in the swings outside the seminary apartments. Mark, who had no children of his own, was impressed with Kathy's vocabulary and asked her, "What is the biggest word you know?" Kathy thought for a moment and then decided "House!"

Mark was amused. He expected some long, sophisticated word. We were pleased that our toddler could think, analyze, and make a decision based on her own observations. To Kathy, the word *biggest* meant large in size. From her perspective there on the swing, our house was the largest thing she could see.

One of the most important skills we can teach our children is the ability to think. We want our sons and daughters to be able to act rationally, identify possibilities, make good choices, and understand consequences. Our children will not benefit from being overly-dependent and attached to their parents when it comes to thinking. We do not want our children to act impulsively, making reckless choices, nor do we want them to act dogmatically, making decisions based on rigid, inflexible positions. We want their decisions to be based on thoughtful consideration and their actions to reflect such a thoughtfulness. As Proverbs 27:12 says, "A prudent man sees danger and hides himself, but the simple go on and suffer for it."

Unfortunately, parents who say that they want their children to grow up into wise decision-makers often do things to stifle thinking during the child's early years. They decide what clothes their child will wear and how their child will spend free time and allowance. They make the child feel that his or her opinions and wishes are wrong or unimportant. Parents can be quick to find fault and to criticize. They become their child's problem-solver, always ready to provide solutions and suggestions; always ready to take over the completion of projects when their child asks for help. While parent's energies would be better invested in teaching conflict resolution skills to their children, they are often tempted to function as a referee in their children's disagreements. They impose their value judgments, deny discussion, and make little effort to consider the validity of the child's point of view. They say, "Don't argue with me. When you've lived as long as I have, maybe you'll understand. For now, you'll do what I say."

Parents do not behave this way because they are unloving. Their actions might be saying, "I don't want you to have to go through the painful experiences I had to face. I want the best for you, and I truly believe that this way is the best." But insisting that children conform to parents' beliefs and authority can backfire. Children can end up feeling powerless and alienated, depending on parents to come to their rescue. Their desire and ability to think for themselves may never grow.

Some parents may say, "If we give our children all the facts they need, they will be prepared to make good decisions." Such parents concentrate on the quantity of information their children can accumulate. But knowing the facts is not enough. Management experts who consult with large businesses agree that the decision-making process is a cycle or loop, not just a one-step action. All decisions, whether complex or simple, involve—

• becoming conscious of a problem,

• investigating the relevant facts and alternatives,

• analyzing the potential consequences,

• choosing and implementing an action, and

• evaluating the result to see if you have addressed the original problem.

Information gathering is only a part of this, not the conclusion.

It is one thing to have the necessary information and quite another to decide how we are going to act upon that information. What we know has to work into our attitudes and our desires. We have to believe that the facts are true for *us*, not just for most people. We must have not only the skills and abilities to make concrete choices, but also the desire to put energy and effort behind that choice. We must be convinced that the probable end results of the decision are results with which we can live.

Our role as parents is to assist our children in being able to recognize problems or issues. We want to make sure that they know how and where to look for relevant information and that they be able to think about the meaning of that information. We want them to be able to act upon their decisions and to be free to evaluate how relevant or successful those actions were. We want them eventually to be able to do all of this on their own! We will probably not be there to help with the decision-making process when our daughters are persuaded with, "If you love me, you'll let me." We will not be the ones to decide if our children are ready to handle the consequences of sexual involvement. We cannot be sure that our sons will practice self-control. These are personal decisions and actions that must be made by individuals. Parents can influence the outcome, but they must do it early by cultivating decision-making competence in their sons and daughters.

Ideas for Helping Children to Think

What specific things can parents do to help their children learn to think for themselves? We can encourage our children to be observant. As we read a picture book together, we can say, "Can you name everything you see on this page?" As we go for a walk, we can stop to watch an ant and guess what plans it has for the bread crumb it carries. We can lie on the grass with our eyes closed and attempt to identify all of the sounds we hear. Neglecting to be alert, we fail to notice so much of life. When we are making decisions, we cannot afford to miss important data. It pays to pay attention!

Children can learn to be aware of what is happening in their environment. They can also learn to check on the *accuracy* of what they observe. Are things really as they appear to be? Did others see the same thing, or something different? What happens if you look at it from a different angle?

A fun way to help your family practice this kind of thinking is by playing object games. Select a variety of objects (almost anything will do), and place them on the table. Ask your children to observe the items carefully for a few minutes, noting as many details as they can. Then, remove or cover the objects, and take turns asking questions to see how observant each person was. "How many buttons were on the bear's shirt? What color was the pencil?" A second object game is to place a selection of objects on the table and again ask your family to observe them carefully. Then, while the children cover their eyes, remove several of the items and change the position of a few of the remaining ones. Then ask your family to open their eyes and identify what is different. A third game is to place objects in a large grocery bag and challenge your children to identify the objects by touch. Ask them to describe the items by their physical characteristics. "Is it rough? Is it hard? Does it feel like it is made of plastic?" These games encourage children to use their senses, to make distinctions, and to give careful thought to their decisions.

Another way to teach your children to think is to ask them to make comparisons—to see similarities and differences and to identify the relationship of one thing or activity to another. "How is the family on your favorite TV show like our family? How is it different? Would you like to be more like them, or should they be more like us? How are older children different from younger children? In what ways are the boys in your class different from the girls? In what ways are they the same?"

We can also encourage thinking by asking our children why they believe something has occurred, or what they think might be a possible solution to a problem. For example, when a lamp gets broken, parents could sit their children down and ask: "How do you think this happened? How can we keep it from happening again?" This is a more productive alternative to angrily scolding, "I've told you a thousand times not to play baseball in the living room!" This kind of thinking helps your children to see that there are consequences to actions and that they often have the power to affect those consequences by their decisions. When your children are fighting over fast-food restaurants, you can say, "Maybe it would be better if Daddy chose tonight" or "Perhaps we should each take turns in choosing." Instead of saying, "That's it! We're never eating out again!" You might propose possible solutions, helping children to see alternatives and building their relational skills.

As we guide our children in learning to make decisions, we must allow them the right to criticize, analyze, and evaluate. Parents are understandably afraid of this. It hurts when a child says, "Mom that dress makes you look fat," and we tend to lash out with some statement about how children should treat their parents with respect. Children *should* respect their parents, and they have no right to say mean and hurtful things. But, making critical judgments is a part of the thinking process. It is a step in assigning worth or determining value. Criticizing seems to come easily; stating the reasoning behind our evaluation is more difficult. A more productive response might be, "Why does it make me look fat? Is it the color, or the design? Is it too small?" We need to teach our children to use the word "because." Show them how important it is to have a valid reason behind their opinions, so evaluating does not degenerate into indiscriminate faultfinding.

Discovering and Claiming Values

With every decision, we are either acting upon or discovering a personal value. Our choices are directed by the things we prize the most. Our decisions, in turn, identify the beliefs that we hold most dear. Once we have recognized our value system, we can begin consciously to organize our lives around that system.

It is not always easy to pinpoint our values. Our vague feelings about them often lead to confusion. "How can I know what is good? I don't know how I feel about that issue. What criteria shall I use to make my decision?" Part of a parent's job is to help children form a value system. This does not mean that parents have to imprint all of their own likes and dislikes onto their children, but they can help their sons and daughters choose, recognize, and claim personal values for themselves.

Young children have values, even when they are not able to state them. They value security and so prefer to stay close to mother. They may refuse to sit in a high chair because they value being part of the family and want to sit on a regular chair at the table like everyone else. Older children can begin to identify their values. Parents can help in this process by frequently asking them, "Would you like to do this?" or "What do you think about that?" Some sample questions parents might use to encourage children to consider their values could be:

—Would you like to buy an ice cream cone or save your money for a toy?

—Would you rather be a great athlete, a great scientist, or a famous comedian?

—Would you rather go to the beach or to the amusement park?

—Do you want to get married?

—What makes you angry?

—If someone gave you ten million dollars, what would you do with it?

—What is the best book you've read this month?

—What has been the happiest moment in your life?

—If you could invite some television characters to your birthday party, whom would you invite?

—What is the worst day of the week for you?

These kinds of questions encourage children to consider and identify what is important and meaningful in their lives. Parents who listen carefully to the answers will be able to help their children note what values are demonstrated. Together the adult and child can set goals and make choices based on those values—choices which we hope will provide deep and lasting satisfaction. We are not suggesting that parents should grill their children with questions. These can be lighthearted discussion topics for the supper table. In fact, sociologists have found that around the supper table is where parents most often talk about their own values!

It is only normal that parents should want their children to share many of their values. But before children decide whether they wish to claim these values for themselves, they must understand the meaning of these values for their own lives. Parents should not assume that children are clear about parents' values. We must talk with our children about the things we stand for, explain why we hold that viewpoint, and demonstrate how we use our values.

For example, churchgoing parents may assume that their daughters and sons know that kindness is a Christian value, then become upset when their youngsters are selfish or mean. Such parents need to explain why they feel loving actions are essential. They will also want to demonstrate love and thoughtfulness in their own actions. Parents should thank their children for acts of kindness and should praise them for thoughtful and considerate behavior. Parents can tell how sad they felt when someone made fun of them or purposely broke their favorite childhood toy. They can invite their children to remember specific situations where unkind behavior caused hurt feelings. They can acquaint their children with Bible passages (such as I Corinthians 13) that stress the value of loving actions.

Parents may mistakenly *assume* that in not talking about premarital intercourse, they are communicating to their children that they believe such behavior is wrong. In fact, the children might be getting the message that *silence* on the topic is what parents value. Parents may then become angry, hurt, ashamed, and confused when their teenager becomes pregnant. Parents need to make sure that they have communicated their actual beliefs to their children and have explained why they feel strongly about the issue. They can explain that premarital intercourse goes against their moral code and violates their religious beliefs. Parents can talk about their own teen years, about the joyful experiences they had in high school, and about how sad it would have been to miss out on those memories because of an unplanned baby. They can discuss how difficult it is to support a family and explain the reasons that many people choose to earn a degree or be settled in a job before having a child. Parents can talk about how many single, unwed mothers live in poverty right here in the United States. Parents can talk about their belief that every child deserves enough food to eat, a warm place to sleep, and the love of two parents.

With this kind of communication, parents are sharing an important part of themselves with their child. They are holding up a value and offering it as a good choice for their child. They are not forcing the value upon their son or daughter, but are enabling him or her to see and understand the validity of that opinion.

How Do You Teach Self-Control

Most parents include self-discipline among the long-term hopes they have for their children. We want to raise daughters and sons who are capable of directing and controlling their own behavior—not just so they will "stay out of trouble," but so they will be able to find personal happiness and success.

How does one go about teaching self-control? If parents pressure a child to behave in a certain way, the control is coming from the outside, not from within the child. Such a child may say, "I'd do it if I could, but my mean Mom won't let me! I wish I were grown up, so I could do what I please!" At the same time, if adults never put outside restraints on a child, it is unlikely that an inner discipline will develop to keep that child from being unruly and out of control. Proverbs 25:28 says, "A man without self-control is like a city broken into, left without walls."

Children need some boundaries to prevent them from harming themselves and others. Surveys show that most accidents to children in the home occur in the late afternoon when parents are tired and preoccupied with preparing supper. Other recent studies indicate that people who are allowed to be bullies as children grow up to be adult bullies. Being given the freedom to do whatever one wants does not usually result in self-control! Self-discipline, then, is not an inherent trait—it must be learned.

The first steps in helping children to learn self-control should begin when children are young. Build their self-esteem so that they are strong and resilient. Help children to respect themselves. Then, communicate to them your values and ethics, providing them with a basis for forming their own goals and expectations for behavior. Teach them to think and make decisions. Give them opportunities to make choices. Be available to listen and assist as they work through those choices.

Next, expect your children to take responsibility for their actions. Let them know that when you say "No" it is for a good reason and that you mean what you say. Don't always bail them out of predicaments or try to cover up their mistakes. Teach them that there are natural or expected consequences to some actions and that we have to live with those consequences.

Another important element in teaching about self-control is making sure that we model self-control in our actions. Children copy behaviors! In our home, for example, the children readily observe that neither mother nor father places a high value on having an uncluttered environment. Our children are aware that when their parents are involved in an exciting project, they do not make housework a priority. It is little wonder, then, that when we decide to clean house, our kids protest and complain! They have not learned self-discipline with regards to always keeping their rooms clean because their parents are undisciplined in this area.

Timmy and Kathy do see us going to the library to do research. They observe the hours we spend planning and preparing for sermons or workshops. They watch us go over a manuscript word by word, editing and rewriting. They see how much we love to read. As a result, we are not surprised that they take responsibility to get their homework done without our prodding. Seeing Mom practicing the piano everyday, our children take for granted that they will practice too. It becomes part of our daily routine and our self-discipline.

If we want our children to exercise self-control in eating habits, use of drugs, or sexual activity, we should model that same discipline ourselves. The success rate of such modeling has been verified by a Swedish study done in 1973. The study showed that when parents told their children to exhibit self-discipline, but did not model that self-control themselves, their instructions were ineffective. But when parents were well-disciplined in an area, their children showed high rates of self-control in that same area. This took place despite the fact that these parents seldom spoke about the need for discipline with their children.

As parents model self-control, as they provide the external discipline that they hope will be internalized, and as they talk with their children about self-discipline, they are helping the child to develop a conscience. The process cannot be forced. We help our children by setting clear goals and expectations, by rewarding positive behavior, and by praising their efforts and successes. Strict parental rules and harsh punishment tend to be ineffective methods for enhancing self-control. They are more likely to produce resentment and hostility than integrity and conscience.

One of the biblical accounts which best exemplifies self-control is the story of Paul and Silas and the earthquake. Arrested, beaten, and humiliated for the "crime" of casting out an evil spirit, the two men found themselves locked and chained in prison. About midnight, while they were singing hymns of praise and praying to God, a great earthquake struck the prison. The earthquake opened the doors, loosened their chains, and Paul and Silas were free.

Paul and Silas might have interpreted the broken chains and open doors as God's signal to escape.

However, they realized that for them to leave the prison would most certainly have caused their jailer to lose his job or even his life. In a remarkable show of self-control, they remained where they were. When the jailer returned, expecting to find his prisoners gone, he was astonished to find them still there. He so admired their courage and inner strength that he asked how he might become more like them. The example of self-control demonstrated by Paul and Silas led to the baptism of the jailer and his entire family.

While we hope that our sons and daughters will never have to face beatings and prison as did Silas and Paul, we know that they will face other threats. They will need to make many choices—choices that will require strong inner values and self-control.

Learning How to Say "No"

When parents hear the statistics for teenage drug abuse, alcoholism, and pregnancy, they become frightened—and rightfully so. They know that their sons and daughters are being pressured to experiment with alcohol, drugs, and sex; and parents wonder, "Will they be able to say 'No'?" Parents of younger children hear stories about child molesters and worry: "Will my children realize that they have the right to tell an adult: 'Don't touch me'?"

A necessary part of good parenting is training our children to be assertive. Assertive behavior means acting in ways to preserve one's dignity and self-respect. Our children need to have faith in themselves and to know that they can stand up for their rights. We must assure them that friends and family members do not always have to agree, that strong relationships can survive disagreements, and that they have the right to say "No" without giving excuses or justifying their reasons!

Many children do not realize that people can, and sometimes will, attempt to use emotional manipulation on them. Young children are taught to respect their parents and other adults and are scolded when they don't obey. They are trained to be obedient and polite and are accustomed to letting others decide how they will act, think, or feel. Boys and girls can be intimidated by another person's apparent logic and may feel foolish or ignorant if they don't go along with that person's desires.

There will be occasions when children of all ages will need to stand up for themselves, either to protect their rights or their bodies. We are giving our children a good gift when we tell them, "You can make your own decisions and stick to them—even when your friends are pushing you to change your mind. I trust your judgment, and you should too." Children can be taught to be persistent. They can learn how to remain firm in their position without becoming angry or hostile and without feeling anxious and guilty.

An excellent book on assertiveness which we recommend is *Yes, I Can Say No—A Parent's Guide To Assertiveness Training For Children*, by Manuel J. Smith (Arbor House, 1986). In this book, Smith outlines "Assertive Rights" that both adults and children have: the right to be your own judge and to be responsible for your thoughts, feelings, and actions; the right to act without making excuses for your behavior and saying, "it's not my fault;" the right to change your mind and to admit making a mistake or to say, "I don't know;" the right to choose your friends; the right to make a decision without having to prove it's logic; the right to say, "I don't understand;" the right to be less than perfect and still feel okay about yourself. Smith's book contains 94 sample dialogs that show how children can give assertive responses to real-life situations. Families can read these dialogs to hear what assertive answers sound like and can roleplay similar situations to practice making their own assertive responses.

David and Bathsheba Should Have Said "No"

As Bible stories so often point out, adults do not always act as they should. King David, for example, made some poor decisions with regards to sex. He spied on Bathsheba while she was bathing. Drawn to her beauty, David allowed his desire to control his actions and sought a way to get around the fact that she was already married. What happened to David's self-control? Why was he not able to say "No" to his desires? Did he never learn self-discipline? What was his understanding of sexual responsibility?

What about Bathsheba? Did she feel she had no right or power to say "No" to David's intentions? Could she have been assertive? Would it have been possible for her to refuse David's wishes?"

When Bathsheba became pregnant with David's child, David arranged to have her husband Uriah come home from battle for the night, hoping to make it appear that the child was Uriah's. But the plan did not work, and David finally resorted to having Uriah sent to the front lines, where he was killed.

David's actions had an effect on himself, on his nation, and on his family. The child conceived by David and Bathsheba died shortly after birth, leaving David feeling depressed and guilty. How differently the story might have ended if David had thought through the possible consequences of his actions and said, "With God's help, I will say no." How differently the story might have ended if women of that day had been raised to think of themselves as equals and not possessions to be used. How much better our own lives and the lives of our children will be when we too can be assertive and comfortable with the word "No."

A Prayer For Clarity of Thought:

Loving God, help us to raise thoughtful children—not just thoughtful in terms of being caring and kind but as persons who are able to think.

Free us from wanting to keep our children overly dependent on us. Help us to enable our sons and daughters to make wise decisions and choices and to have the ability to carry out the actions they decide upon.

Help us to communicate our values and our love for you, to practice self-control in our own lives, and to be assertive in our "Yes" and in our "No." Amen.

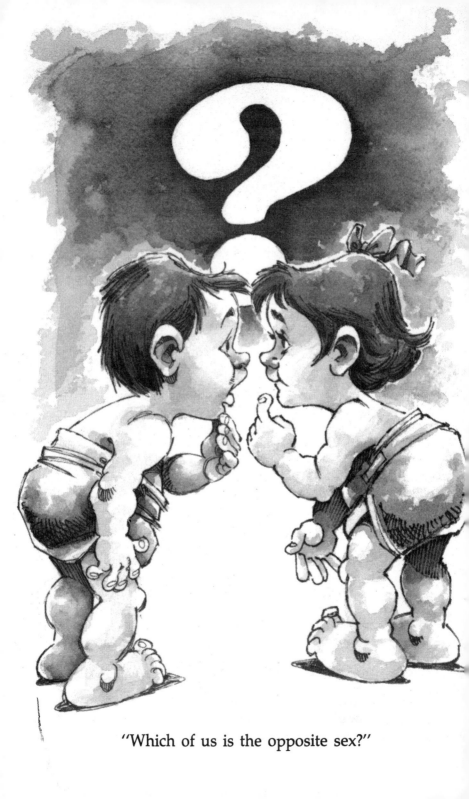

"Which of us is the opposite sex?"

CHAPTER 3

UNDERSTANDING OUR CHILDREN'S SEXUALITY

Becoming Aware of Our Sexuality

Can you remember when you first realized that you were a boy or a girl? Most adults cannot. As infants, we neither knew nor cared about such differences—even though people made a fuss over what a beautiful girl or strong and husky boy we were.

Over the next two years, we frequently heard these comments. We began to notice that boys and girls dressed differently and observed that our mother and father did not have identical hairstyles. We might have observed that Brother or Sister did not urinate in the same way we did. By the time we were two and a half or three years old, we were able to say with certainty, "No, I am *not* a girl" or "No, I am *not* a boy." We were able to identify our own sex and the sex of others with reasonable accuracy.

The process by which children become aware of their sexuality is a gradual one, occurring in predictable stages. This does not mean that infants are asexual or without sexuality, for every person, regardless of age, is a sexual being. Infants might not be able to label their gender, but they are sexual from the moment of birth. Sexuality is an integral part of every person's identity.

Some adults feel uncomfortable with the idea that children are sexual beings. "How can someone this innocent and pure be called sexual?" They do not want children to demonstrate sexual behaviors or knowledge. Observing children engaging in an activity which they see as sexual, they become upset.

We are not suggesting that parents should simply ignore or laugh off a child's inappropriate sexual behaviors. It is a parent's responsibility to help children form strong values and to communicate the difference between appropriate and inappropriate behavior. As adults, we have learned much about life and relationships, both from personal experiences and often from the guidance of our own parents. We know that issues of sexuality hold the potential for both joy and pain, and we feel an obligation to make sure our children are aware of possible danger areas. In keeping with the wisdom of the psalmist,

> things we have heard and known,
> things that our fathers told us.
> We will not keep them from our children.
> Psalm 78:3-4

We do not want our children to be hurt by unnecessary mistakes. We try to pass on our values. We intend for them to be a positive guide for our children, but at times end up judging children by adult standards. We scold them or punish their innocent and natural actions because by adult standards such actions appear suggestive. At the same time, we encourage children to act in even *more* suggestive ways by rationalizing that she will look so cute or that he will look all grown up. As parents we may fail to recognize our inconsistency in response to children's sexuality.

When our daughter Kathryn was in kindergarten, she participated in a dancing and gymnastics class. For the spring recital, each little girl was expected to purchase two sequined outfits. The day of the recital, these five- and six-year-olds spent the entire afternoon rolling their hair in electric rollers and cementing the curls on the top of their heads with hair spray and hundreds of bobby pins. The make-up crew sculpted the girls' faces with blush, eye shadow, mascara, and lipstick. When nervous tears made the make-up run, more was liberally applied to hide the evidence. At the close of the show, everyone said what beautiful young ladies they were! No one said, "My, how sexy you looked," but that was the implied message.

The following afternoon, several of these little dancers were taken to the park to play. It was a hot, humid Texas day, and most of the girls were wearing short sundresses. One small girl, praised on the previous evening for looking so appealing, began to turn cartwheels and stand on her head, giving full view of her underpants. Her mother, dressed in short shorts and a halter top, rushed over to give her daughter a swat on her behind. "Nice little girls don't show their underwear!" she scolded. "Especially with boys around!"

There is nothing inherently wrong in wanting our daughters to be feminine. Some five- and six-old girls may already have a desire to look pretty. For such girls, this desire may be natural. Other equally normal children do not share their interest. However, for pre-pubescent girls to spend hours "becoming beautiful" is probably not natural or even healthy. On the other hand, it *is* developmentally normal for a small child to try to stand on her head. Little girls at this age don't usually think, "It would be sexy to let a boy see my underwear, so I think I'll turn a cartwheel!" Six-year-olds turn cartwheels for the joy of it.

Sequences of Sexual Development

Although every person is unique, there appear to be sequences of sexual development that are similar for most children. As children pass through these sequences, we are reminded that it is important for children to be children in all areas of development, including sexual development. As I Corinthians 13:11a says: "When I was a child, my speech, feelings, and thinking were all those of a child." The passage goes on to say that when we become adults, we put away childish things; but it does not say, "So don't ever act like a child" or "Childhood is not as good as adulthood" or "Children should behave as miniature adults." Each step of development represents a stage that should be affirmed as a part of God's creative plan. Our appreciation can echo the words of the psalmist:

> You created every part of me;
>   you put me together in my mother's womb.
> I praise you because you are to be feared;
>   all you do is strange and wonderful.
> I know it with all my heart.
>   Psalm 139:13-14

At each age level there are ways in which boys and girls tend to differ, as well as numerous parallels in their behaviors. While some of these similarities and differences may be biological in origin, others are culturally-induced. Frequently, the actual cause is difficult to distinguish. Research findings in the area of developmental differences have often been challenged by conflicting data.

The information that follows details sexual development and the corresponding parent support that is appropriate for five age levels.

BEFORE BIRTH

Stages In Sexual Development

Sexual development begins long before birth. From the moment of fertilization, when the father's sperm contributes either an X or Y chromosome to pair with the X chromosome of the mother's ovum, the cells of boys and girls are slightly different. The male cell contains an X chromosome and a smaller Y chromosome (XY), while the female cell contains two large X chromosomes (XX).

John Money of Johns Hopkins University is one of many authorities who believe that both maternal and fetal hormones also affect the development of body gender.[1] Hormones—biochemical substances that are present in the blood in minute amounts—determine the kind of external sex organs an embryo will develop. Up until about the sixth week after conception, or possibly as late as the twelfth week for females, the tissue structures that will become the female or male reproductive organs are the same. Unless male hormones are present, a female body is formed. Hormones, then, appear to be responsible for the visible differences between females and males.

Other prenatal chemical adjustments are also believed to have an effect on the sex of a fetus. For example, barbituates taken by pregnant women have been found to prevent the male sex organs from developing properly—a continuing reminder of the problems caused by drug abuse.

Sexual identity is not established at conception, nor is it determined during the months in the womb. Hundreds of factors in a person's childhood environment will help to shape his or her personality. However, the prenatal months have a great influence as the genetic blueprint is laid down and then as hormonal activity occurs. These will serve as the foundation for later physical, mental, and sexual development.

Providing a Solid Basis For Children's Sexuality

Expectant parents who want to provide a solid basis for their child's sexuality start by obtaining good prenatal care and by avoiding the use of drugs, alcohol, and tobacco. Medical research has shown that these can be extremely harmful to the fetus. Loving your child, even before birth, increases the possibility of that child forming a positive self-image in the future. Such actions are stepping stones to the eventual awareness that loving actions bring loving responses.

BIRTH THROUGH ONE YEAR OF AGE

Differences Between Boys and Girls

In a study conducted by S. B. Gurvity and K. A. Dodge in 1975, a videotape of an infant was shown to mothers and fathers of young babies who were to analyze the child's behavior. The baby was dressed so that viewers could not tell whether it was a boy or a girl.

BIRTH—1 YEAR

When the men were told that the baby was a female, they were more likely to say positive things about the infant—characterizing her as gentle, less aggressive, sweet, a soft crier, and sociable. When the men were told that this same baby was a boy, they tended to describe the baby as fussy, irritable, and aggressive. The women, on the other hand, were more likely to respond positively to the baby when told it was a boy. They would assign to the child traditional masculine attributes, describing the baby as strong, active, and independent. The women would characterize this same infant less favorably when told it was a girl. Many of these impressions of maleness and femaleness are qualities we see when we *look* for them, rather than being actual distinctions. At the same time, some sex-related differences do exist between baby boys and girls—many of which are either proven or well-supported by most published studies.

First of all, more males are conceived than females, with approximately 106 boys born in the United States for every 100 girls. But the percentage of miscarriages and the infant mortality rate are higher for males than for females. The death rate within the first month after birth is nearly 25 percent higher for males than for females. Boys are more susceptible to hereditary disorders, disease, and malnutrition at all ages, and the disproportionate ratio of male to female deaths continues throughout life. By age fifteen, the number of boys and girls in the United States is approximately equal.[2]

At birth, boys are heavier than girls, with larger heads and faces, more muscle, and less fat. Baby girls are physically more mature than boys. They learn to walk earlier and tend to cut teeth sooner. Girls are more sensitive to touch, pain, cold, and taste than boys are. Some studies show that boys startle more easily than girls, cry more frequently, and are more difficult to soothe. Infant boys and girls also have different sleep patterns.

The right side of the brain, which is considered responsible for processing language, develops earlier in females than in males. Girls, then, frequently talk earlier and excel in verbal activities. Some studies have indicated that infant girls can recognize faces at an earlier age than infant boys. By six months of age, girls show more interest in fixing their eyes on pictures of human faces. They begin to smile before boys do and are more easily encouraged to smile.

BIRTH—1 YEAR

Stages In Sexual Development

Both male and female infants show evidence of sexual response. Infant boys have erections—often during a diaper change. Males experience erections prior to birth and are sometimes born with an erection. Females, prior to birth and as infants, experience vaginal lubrication and orgasmic responses.

As infants gain command of their muscles, they begin to move their arms and reach out for things. At approximately sixteen weeks, babies' hands are at their mouths. At twenty weeks they move their hands and arms in the area of the chest. By the fortieth week they are beginning to explore in the area of the thighs and genitals. As babies make significant advances in their self-discovery, they play with the navel and touch the penis or vulva. In some ways, the baby's own body is just one of the many things that infants grasp and manipulate. But babies also discover that touching their genitals results in a pleasurable sensation, which may be the onset of masturbation. Early in life both sexes experience feelings that are directly related to their being female or male.

Actions such as making eye contact (at four weeks), smiling at the sight of a mother's face (at eight weeks), crying when someone leaves (at twenty weeks), or withdrawing from strangers (at 32 weeks), all show how babies are beginning the process of relating to others. This has sexual implications, because establishing an intimate relationship with another person is part of what sexuality is all about.

One of the major ways that infants respond to and communicate with others is through the sense of touch. Babies feel warmth and affection when Daddy plays with them. They usually like to be cuddled. When babies nurse, they not only experience physical pleasure but are also nourished by the security and comfort of their mother's body. They sense nervousness or fear by the way they are held, and are aware of the holder's emotional state. Babies' cries are pleas for comfort. They welcome being picked up, rubbed gently on the tummy or the back, or rocked to sleep. Such quiet touches are calming and help children to initiate control on their own.

Less than seventy years ago, childhood authorities encouraged parents to avoid spoiling their babies with too much handling. Parents were told to let babies cry, to feed them on an exact schedule, and to avoid overusing the rocking chair or cradle. Babies, parents were told, should not be smothered with touch. Today we know that physical touch is essential in order for a baby to thrive.

BIRTH—1 YEAR

Touch influences learning, growth rates, sociability, the ability to withstand stress, and even immunological development. Infants who are not touched experience setbacks in growth. They may have speech defects, mental retardation, decreased height and weight, and are sometimes said to have "psychosocial dwarfism." Persons who are not held and fondled may suffer later in life from either an extreme hunger for body contact or an intense repulsion to touch. Researchers Mary Ainsworth[3] and M. Louise Biggar[4] have also found that infants who are physically rejected by their mothers in the first three months of life will show unusually high degrees of anger by the time they are a year old.

It has been found that massaging babies' backs may help them build a healthy body image and improve their neurological development. Holding and touching infants helps them to stay healthy, increases their skin's sensitivity to stimulus, and enhances their socialization skills. Dr. Anneliese F. Korner[5] has discovered that picking up crying newborn babies and holding them close to the shoulder almost invariably causes the infant to become bright-eyed and alert. Babies who are alert have more opportunities to relate to the people and the environment which they see. When a baby is only soothed and not lifted to the shoulder, there is no significant increase in visual alertness. Early contact—touching an infant within thirty minutes after birth—results in significantly stronger bonding attachments between parent and child. These early-held children cry less and smile and laugh more than babies who are not cuddled immediately after birth.

Touch, then, is an essential ingredient in a small child's sexual development. It encompasses and enhances so many areas of that sexuality—the ability to relate intimately with another person and to be sensitive to their needs and emotions; the ability to experience pleasurable sensations and to feel good about one's own body; and the ability to accept, appreciate, and reciprocate physical and emotional tenderness from special individuals.

Psychologist Erik Erikson[6] suggests that during the first year of life, babies are learning to trust themselves and others. This too has an impact on children's experience of sexuality. When babies feel safe and confident, they become free to reach out past themselves and to feel secure in accepting the love of others. Trust enables persons to disclose themselves to someone they love—an important step on the way to becoming vulnerable and open in relationships.

BIRTH—1 YEAR

Providing a Solid Basis for Children's Sexuality

Parents can help their newborn children have a good start on attaining a positive sexuality by doing their best to help them thrive. We can give our tiny sons every chance to survive that statistically difficult first month. We can provide good medical care and proper nutrition. Mothers can choose to breastfeed their babies, knowing that human milk provides the best nutrition possible for the child. Breast milk is more easily digested than cow's milk. The colostrum in the mother's milk provides antibodies which protect the baby against disease. Breastfeeding is also an ideal opportunity for the mother-child closeness which is so critical to early bonding. In instances where breastfeeding is either not possible or not desired, parents can still hold and cuddle their babies during feedings and at other times.

It is natural for parents to become frustrated and overwhelmed at times—especially when they are exhausted. Remember that many little girls dislike being cold and many little boys cry a lot. Our children are not trying to upset us. If we respond to children with anger and irritation, they will sense it, even if they do not yet understand our feelings. Treating tiny children as if they are doing something wrong when they really can't help how they are acting may lead to a negative self-image later in life.

Remember the importance of loving, warm, gentle touches. We can cuddle our babies, massage their backs, make eye contact as we talk to them. Instead of always leaving them in a crib or infant seat, we can hold them upright on our shoulder and let them see the world. When our babies begin to discover different parts of their bodies, we should not slap their hands because of our own embarrassment. The way we hold and touch our children can assure them that we are persons they can trust. Our building trust in our children will help them later to form the intimate bonds and ties that will make other relationships possible.

BIRTH—1 YEAR

ONE AND TWO YEARS OF AGE

Differences Between Boys and Girls:

During the next two years of life, differences between girls and boys become evident. Boys show more hostility and anger than girls, even by as early as seven months of age, and the differences

1 AND 2 YEARS

are often sizable by the age of two or two and a half. Many boys engage in highly rough-and-tumble play, and although girls frequently do so in moderate ways, research suggests that about 20 percent of boys are much rougher than any of the girls.

Difference in play style shows itself in the use of toys. Boys appear to play with trucks and cars more than girls, even though small children are much more likely to see their mothers driving the family car. Parents may offer children identical toys, yet find that boys and girls choose and play with those toys in dissimilar ways. A study in modern Israel found that most parents gave dolls to their toddlers. While the girls tended to play with their dolls as imitation babies, the boys might jump on the dolls or pound with them as if they were hammers.

Surprisingly, evidence does not show that little boys are encouraged to be more aggressive than little girls. Parents and nursery workers appear to be more aware of boys' aggression and quicker to discourage it, while they tend to ignore the aggressive behavior of girls. Some researchers believe that the source of male aggression is hormonal. Studies have found that hormonal treatments can make female animals behave as aggressively as males. Researchers Carol Jacklin and Eleanor Maccoby[7] of Stanford University believe that boys are genetically more *prepared* to become aggressive—not inherently aggressive, but requiring only small amounts of stimulation to bring out aggression.

Another sex-related difference observed in toddlers is the degree of cooperation. In an experiment by L. Shapio[8] at Harvard University, previously unacquainted two-year-olds were brought together in pairs. When a single toy was placed between the children, the pairs of boys would treat one another suspiciously, evaluate each other's posture and facial expression, then fight over possession of the toy. The pairs of girls appeared to be more trusting of each other playing together cooperatively.

Females, as a group, learn to talk earlier than males. Girls have a larger vocabulary and use grammar and pronunciation more correctly. By two years of age, girls usually know the names of their family and friends. Boys, as a rule, do not. Parents of two-year-old daughters may believe that their little girl is smarter than the neighbor's little boy. Parents of boys can be assured that their sons will soon begin to exhibit their own unique strengths.

1 AND 2 YEARS

Stages In Sexual Development

The sexuality of one- and two-year-old children is being shaped by greater physical skills, emerging independence, increasing self-awareness, social learning, and the beginning of friendship. The psychologist Erikson refers to this as the stage of autonomy or self-determination. Toddlers are no longer insistent or dependent on close contact with mother, but want to walk and run, to explore and manipulate the world. When mother makes suggestions and demands, the average 21-month-old obeys only about half of the time. Children of this age are becoming aware of their own wants and are building their self-esteem and self-identity. Parents' punishments may cause feelings of shame and doubt.

Toddlers are beginning to want companionship. These companions are often family members—parents, brothers, and sisters. Sometimes ones and twos will actively play with another person, but they may be satisfied simply to have another person close by.

One- and two-year-olds are interested in the human body. By age two, many toddlers recognize photographs of themselves as well as their own image in a mirror. By two and a half, children refer to themselves as "I" and to others as "you." They begin to notice differences between the sexes—differences in bodies and differences in the ways those bodies are dressed. At this age children state their sex negatively—"I am not a boy" or "I am not a girl." They watch curiously when others are undressed. They are conscious of their genitals and may handle them.

One- and two-year-olds learn about life by observing and imitating. Children watch, compare, and copy behaviors—especially the actions of their parents, adopting behaviors that produce rewards. With this process, children begin to learn skills and attitudes that are essential for living in society. Pressures are put upon children to do things in a sex-appropriate way, starting with the play materials that are offered to them and the clothes in which they are dressed.

One of the major tasks of a toddler is to begin toilet training. Parents' attitudes towards this training will probably affect the child's feelings about sex, simply because the same body parts are involved. Taught that it is dirty to urinate or to have a bowel movement, they may conclude that sex also is dirty. If children receive criticism about their lack of control, they may feel tension or

1 AND 2 YEARS

shame in relation to these body parts. Parents who are uncomfortable using the correct names of body parts during toilet training have difficulty talking openly and candidly about sex when the child is older.

Providing a Solid Basis for Children's Sexuality

Parents of toddlers can build a solid basis for their children's sexuality by providing a variety of toys for both sexes. Parents must then be willing to accept children's choice of toys and how they choose to enjoy them—even when their choices are not consistent with traditional images of little girl or little boy behaviors.

We should probably not expect a rough and tumble boy to be quiet and subdued all the time. We can give him a doll or bear to cuddle, but we do not want to make him feel that it is bad to be active. When our son is behaving in ways which we feel are too aggressive, however, we don't ignore it. If he wants to pound and starts to use a doll as the hammer, we can give him the proper toys. This does not mean we take away the doll. We talk about how babies need love and like to be held and hugged and how hammers are for pounding and for building. We give little boys an opportunity to use their muscles and still let them know that hurting people is not something we do, even in fun or imaginary play.

We train children in positive sexuality by teaching cooperation. Sharing is a difficult concept for a child to learn. Yet, a truly intimate relationship with another person is impossible without sharing yourself. We need to teach our sons and daughters to trust and to expect the best of their companions. The Bible records several stories about sharing. 1 Samuel 18 tells how Jonathan gave his own weapons and clothing to David as a sign of friendship. Acts 2 recalls how early Christians shared everything they owned. The story of Ruth in the Old Testament tells how Boaz was willing to share his crops with Ruth and Naomi. Sharing is indeed a value that we want our children to embrace.

What else can parents do to enhance toddlers' sexuality? We can allow them to have some independence and can provide playmates. We can be relaxed and unembarrassed in our method of toilet training. We can let them see that their parents care deeply for them and for one another. Husbands and wives can still hold hands when they walk down the beach. Sadly, surveys conducted by University of Minnesota researchers at shopping malls, on the beach, outside the church, and at the zoo show that parents tend not to laugh, smile, or hold hands when accompanied by their children. We can change those statistics!

THREE THROUGH FIVE YEARS OF AGE

Differences Between Boys and Girls

Between the ages of three and five, children are in the process of forming their sexual identity. During these years their gender appears to become fixed, making later changes in sex-role behaviors and attitudes psychologically difficult. Because of this, preschool boys and girls appear to demonstrate many obvious differences, and these differences will probably influence their interests and attitudes for the rest of their lives.

One area of differences is that of play. Although preschool boys and girls still play together, they are beginning to spend more time with children of their own sex and are more likely to fight with a sibling or playmate who is of the opposite sex. Boys tend to play in larger groups than girls do. When given a free choice, boys often choose to play with tricycles, blocks, trucks, cars, and guns. They pretend to be firefighters, airplane pilots, soldiers, or one of their Saturday morning cartoon heroes. A majority of little girls, on the other hand, want to play house with their dolls and pretend to be Mommy. When preschoolers sit down to draw pictures or to tell stories, the little girls include people in their stories and pictures much more frequently than the little boys do.

Preschool boys are slightly heavier and taller than girls of the same age, but girls, on the average, tend to be about six months ahead in general physical, emotional, and social development. Boys' bodies have a higher percentage of muscle and a lower percentage of fat. Their hearts are larger and their circulatory systems are more efficient. Partly for these reasons, boys can become proficient in throwing a ball and in motor skills requiring coordination of many different muscles. They spend more time than girls do in active outdoor play, excelling in activities which require muscularity and stamina such as climbing, wrestling, and running.

3—5 YEARS

Girls usually prefer less strenuous activities, but are better than boys at hopping, skipping, jumping rope, and standing on one foot. Girls also begin to show a superiority in manual dexterity and are better at using scissors and fastening buttons.

As they get older, boys appear to become more adventuresome than girls and to do more exploring. When they have explored near home, boys may want to discover new places. The typical girl stays closer to home. Little boys are more likely to try to pet a strange dog or to climb too high on the playground equipment or to come too close to a deep hole. This may be one reason that they have more accidents than girls do. Researchers believe that girls are not less curious or adventuresome, but are probably subjected to greater restrictions. Parents may be more protective of their daughters and quicker to warn them of possible dangers.

On the other hand, researchers have discovered that even when treated in a similar manner by parents, boys and girls do not always respond in the same way. For example, when parents are authoritative, their daughters appear to increase in independence and their sons appear to be more compliant. It is difficult, then, to determine conclusively why boys and girls act in the ways they do.

Stages in Sexual Development

Three-, four-, and five-year-olds are very interested in babies. "Where does a baby come from? Where is it before it is born?" They often decide that a baby is born through the navel. They ask parents to give them a baby brother or sister, and both boys and girls talk about the babies they will have when they grow up.

Preschoolers have a strong interest in the human body—their own and others. They are concerned with their body build and wonder why some children are tall and thin while others are short and plump. They want to know the names of the body organs and want to talk about their awareness of sex. This is the age when boys and girls are full of curiosity about why and how their bodies differ from those of adults and from children of the opposite sex. They want to see their parents' naked bodies. They touch and explore themselves. They ask to look at the bodies of their friends and willingly show their's in return, examining each other's genitals and watching each other urinate. Such play is natural because it *is* play, a

3—5 YEARS

way in which the child explores the mysterious human body and begins to prepare for adulthood.

Three-, four-, and five-year-olds are aware of their gender and want their appearance to be what they have observed as appropriate for their sex. Little boys sometimes ask to wear ties; little girls like to wear all of their jewelry at once. Choices in hairstyle, clothing, toys, and even colors are made on the basis of being boys or girls. Preschoolers do not appreciate or enjoy being teased about being tomboys or sissies. This is the developmental stage during which children's gender identity is becoming fixed, and the child appears extremely cognizant of sex-role typing. They make strong identifications with the same-sex parent, although they often are not carbon-copies of parental behaviors or attitudes and may even feel jealous over or competitive with that parent.

Providing a Solid Basis for Children's Sexuality

Parents of preschoolers are providing sex education as they answer their children's questions about the human body, sex, and babies with honesty and openness. We can make certain our children have friends of both sexes. If the neighborhood children decide to play doctor, we can remain calm, using it as an opportunity to talk frankly about the human body, rather than condemning such play as evil. We are providing a solid basis for our children's sexuality when we allow them enough choice in the kinds, colors, and textures of clothing they like to wear. This is one way to help them define themselves. We can let our children make choices in other areas too and not demand that they be carbon copies of their parents.

In our family, Timothy is a child who cares very deeply about the clothes he wears. He wants to wear suit jackets on Sundays, even though his father would probably be happy to wear blue jeans and a T-shirt every day. Timothy knows the hairstyle he likes and is bothered when his hair is contrary. His daddy, on the other hand, rarely thinks about hair and is comfortable with the mussed-up look. As parents, we have decided to respect Tim's feelings and wishes concerning his appearance. We try to do our best to keep clean the white jeans he insists on wearing whenever possible and don't expect him to share his dad's opinions on the relative importance of looks. We want him to know that there are many ways to be masculine, not only his father's way. We want him to be himself and to have good feelings when he looks in the mirror. Positive sexuality, we believe, goes hand in hand with positive self-esteem.

SIX THROUGH EIGHT YEARS OF AGE

Differences Between Boys and Girls

When children reach elementary school age, boys are beginning to assume the general body shape of a man with a long, muscular chest and shoulders broader than the hips. Their chests are relatively bigger than girls', and their muscular capacity is about 10 percent greater. Girls are beginning to show feminine distribution of fat, especially around the hips.

First, second, and third grade girls often have a best friend, tending to prefer close one-on-one relationships with another girl. Because they play in pairs, they easily cause and experience jealousy, and friendships are not always long-lasting. Boys tend to play in groups and are less exclusive in their relationships. They also appear to be more competitive in some situations and seem to have more enduring friendships than do the girls.

In 1975, researchers Whiting and Whiting[9] observed children from around the world in their home settings. They discovered that in almost every culture, girls are more apt than boys to help adults and other children. Boys were more likely to seek attention from adults and to attempt to dominate other children, while girls were more pro-social—wanting to help, share, and listen. In another study, researchers held a coloring contest for grade school children in which the children had to share crayons for a color-by-number competition. The result of this study also showed that girls were more likely to share, usually handing over a color when asked to. Boys, however, were less likely to share the requested crayon. Furthermore, they were significantly less likely to share with a friend, as opposed to a mere acquaintance, which may indicate that competition is a major factor between friends.

Boys and girls have been found to be fairly equal in reading and vocabulary competence, although girls tend to show faster verbal development. On the average, grade school girls are still ahead of boys in development. More males (such as children who complete a

6—8 YEARS

college education) have been identified as child geniuses, and there are more boys than girls who are diagnosed as autistic or hyperactive. Boys also have a much higher percentage of learning disabilities.

Stages in Sexual Development

Six-, seven-, and eight-year-old children are still interested in the differences in body structure between boys and girls and may continue to engage in sex play and masturbation. They may begin to fantasize or daydream about sex, but appear to have *less* interest in sex than they did earlier and ask fewer questions. The questions they do ask begin to be more factual, such as "Does it hurt to have a baby?" At six, children are not self-conscious about their bodies, but by the ages of seven or eight a sense of sexual modesty usually appears. They can become easily embarrassed and tend to desire privacy. They are also learning to respect the rights of others.

School-age children have already formed strong ideas about appropriate sex roles. After about the second grade there seems to be no increase in attachment to sexual stereotypes. Although children may think a bit less stereotypically about what is appropriate for a man or a woman, boys remain under pressure to be masculine. Grade school children tend to segregate themselves by sex on the playground and may start to join boys' or girls' clubs.

Children at this age show contradictory social traits. They fight more frequently with best friends and siblings than they do with other children. When someone is hurt, it is often the most aggressive child who displays sympathy for the injury.

Grade school children may delight in off-color jokes or using unacceptable language, even when they may not understand the meaning of what they are repeating. Their attempts to build self-confidence and to establish some independence from adults may explain such behavior, but they are also beginning to form ethical standards of goodness for themselves and others. They can understand that growing up means assuming more responsibility and accepting consequences for one's decisions. They want approval from parents and peers and are beginning to see that love and respect for others presupposes a love of self.

Early elementary children are interested in the development of babies and will still often request that their parents have one. They

6—8 YEARS

can understand the concept that babies need both a father and a mother to be formed and that plants and animals each reproduce their own kind. They are able to compare the development of human babies with the development of animals and can learn about life by observing their pets.

Providing a Solid Basis for Children's Sexuality

One thing parents can do for their first, second, and third grade children is to encourage them to be pro-social—to form friendships and to act in socially responsible ways. Boys and girls do not automatically know how to work with others or know how to care for the needs and feelings of their friends and family members. They may be shy, selfish, or thoughtless—not because they are bad, but because they are immature and because they see their friends acting in these same ways. Children need our support and guidance in these areas, and our praise when they do well. The church and Sunday school can be a major source of this support.

Don remembers an experience he had as a child in which he learned what it means to be pro-social. It was the day of the school picnic. A younger and much smaller boy—who had had a difficult year—came up to Don, hit him, and tried to start a fight. Don just stood there while the boy kept hitting him. Don's friends said, "What's the matter with you? Don't let him do that. Hit him back." Don's teachers said, "What a mature thing to do, to just ignore the boy. We are proud of you." What his teachers said made a lasting impression on Don. He is sure that without the *positive* reinforcement from those adults, the *negative* reinforcement of his peers would have convinced him to fight back. On that afternoon he learned to care for the needs and feelings of another person—a skill that is essential for the formation of a good sexual relationship.

Parents of elementary children provide a solid foundation for their children's sexuality when they help their children to become thoughtful and caring. They help their daughters and sons become well-adjusted in their sexual identity when they determine not to put their children under undue academic pressure by saying, "Your *sister* was reading on a sixth grade level when she was your age" or "Your *brother* was always good at math." Developmental differences can make some subjects and tasks much more difficult for some children than for others. Comparing a child's academic,

6—8 YEARS

6—8 YEARS

musical, athletic, or artistic skills to those of a sibling is neither helpful nor kind.

Parents can continue to answer their children's questions honestly and in the same spirit in which the questions were asked. Pat answers, answers that make light of the issue, or answers that attempt to change the subject are inappropriate responses to questions that may be difficult or personal. Parents can respect their child's need for privacy. They can give their child a pet and discuss the process of reproduction using the pet as an example. Grade school children are usually able to make the connection between what they see in their pets and what happens in human life.

When young grade school children come home with off-color jokes or words, parents can use these jokes and words as teachable moments, turning a potentially upsetting episode into a positive one. The child is not helped when parents act shocked and horrified to hear these words. Neither does it help to give the impression that using such language is cute. Instead, parents can ask children if they understand what the word or joke means and explain any misconceptions. They can discuss why sexual jokes and the use of sex-related profanity can be painful to people. They can help their children find ways other than using sexually aggressive language to express feelings of frustration and anger.

NINE THROUGH TWELVE YEARS OF AGE

Differences Between Boys and Girls

9—12 YEARS

All through childhood, girls are ahead of boys developmentally. The average twelve-year-old girl is taller, heavier, and two years closer to physical maturity than the average twelve-year-old boy. Girls usually experience a marked growth spurt at age ten or eleven, while boys grow more quickly around age twelve or thirteen. Boys continue to demonstrate more strength and physical ability.

One seemingly common characteristic at this age is that in mixed-sex situations, girls usually seem unwilling to compete with boys. For example, studies of children from very different cultural groups found that girls were much less competitive when playing dodge ball against boys than they were when playing against other girls, even when both had equal experience. Some girls, when playing with other girls, were measured to have high playing skills.

But when playing with boys, these girls were likely to stand with their legs crossed and their arms folded, or to talk to one another instead of paying attention to the game. As a result, when playing in mixed-sex games, the boys almost invariably won, even when low-skilled boys played against high-skilled girls.

Boys and girls during this period tend to have larger circles of friends than they did when they were younger. Some are beginning to admire members of the opposite sex, with girls more interested in boys than boys are in girls, but most choose to play and talk with members of their own sex. Girl's relationships often appear to have more complexities, with emotional quarrels, jealousy over sharing friends, and criticism of one another.

By the upper elementary grades, boys may appear to have superior mathematical ability and to do better in visual-spatial activities such as manipulating objects in a three-dimensional space or reading maps. Girls often appear to excel at reading comprehension, vocabulary, and verbal creativity. Research in these areas continues. Some recent studies support the conclusion that these differences are based on ability, while others suggest the cause is cultural expectation and bias.

People have recently begun to discard some traditional but unjustified ideas concerning the difference between boys and girls. Examples of common beliefs that have been disproved are:
— Boys have a greater motivation to achieve
— Girls have a lower self-esteem than boys
— Boys are better at complex tasks
— Girls are better at simple, repetitive tasks
— Boys are less social than girls
— Boys are more responsive to visual stimuli and girls more responsive to what they hear.

Eleanor Maccoby and Carolyn Jacklin[7] after careful review of numerous experimental studies with boys and girls, have concluded that all of the above generalizations are without support.

Stages in Sexual Development

Nine- through twelve-year-olds have an increased interest in sex, although they ask fewer questions than younger children do. Their interests are now kept more private. Masturbation and sex play may occur, but not openly, and young persons who masturbate

9—12 YEARS

frequently may feel worried or guilty about it. Children this age may experience a lot of peer pressure to be able to tell and understand the humor of off-color jokes. They may also be interested in viewing R-rated movies and television shows.

During this pre-adolescent stage, young persons are more likely to talk to friends about sex than to parents. Studies show that while mothers and daughters do talk some, few conversations on sex occur between mothers and sons, fathers and sons, or fathers and daughters. If parents have not modeled an openness to their children's sex-related questions, the children are going to find it difficult to talk about their feelings and may be easily embarrassed.

Since homosexual issues are frequently discussed in current society and particularly since AIDS has become an important health issue, children may be curious about the meaning of homosexuality. They may have misunderstandings and worries, especially if they have had strong feelings toward adults or peers of the same sex or if they have engaged in sex play with same-sex friends. Parents should be prepared to assure their sons and daughters that curiosity about or attraction to people of the same sex is not in itself an indication of homosexuality.

Even as early as eight, nine, or ten, some children may be coming into physical maturity. Some girls will begin to menstruate, and some boys will find that their testicles and penis are becoming larger. Some are beginning to experience body changes such as the growth of pubic hair, the development of breasts, or the deepening of the voice. Boys may begin to have more frequent erections and may experience nocturnal emissions. Some children will resent the physical changes taking place; some will feel self-conscious and embarrassed. Most will look forward to taking on an adult appearance and may be concerned if they lag behind friends in reaching physical maturity.

Recent studies by Sandra Weiss[10] have found that older grade school children still need to be hugged and held by their parents and that parental touch continues to have a direct relationship to the development of a positive body image. When parents—and especially fathers—touch their children in an intentional, loving manner, the result tends to be children who have good feelings about their bodies.

Other studies have found that as children become older, their need to be in close human contact appears to increase. Despite their attempts to reject affection, adolescents need to be touched or cuddled. Being held may promote relaxation, provide a sense of security, and reduce anxiety. Unfortunately, the older children become, the less likely parents are to hold and touch them. Fearing that hugs may be inappropriate or even that they might be rejected, parents may shy away from touching their maturing children. A possible reason behind early sexual activity could be the increasing need that boys and girls have for physical contact and the decreasing availability of such contact in the family.

Older grade school students may be interested in the scientific facts related to sex. They may find it easier to ask personal questions when they are cloaked in general rather than personal terms and may appreciate reading books or leaflets on the subject. They may also be curious about pornography as an alternate source of information, especially if sex is not a subject of open discussion at home. Parents should not overreact to this but can quietly use the discovery of such material as an opportunity to open a discussion.

Providing a Solid Basis for Children's Sexuality

Parents of pre-adolescents see their child growing taller and starting to develop a mature body, and may worry that their son or daughter will grow up too soon. They hear stories of ten-year-old girls giving birth and wonder how much their own child understands about sexual intercourse. There are so many things they want their child to know, yet it seems to be getting more difficult to talk. What can a parent do?

Parents can resist the temptation to tease their sons or daughters about physical changes. Children are very sensitive about their bodies. They are often perplexed and feel self-conscious and unsure of themselves. This does not mean that humor does not have its place. Humor can make conversations about sexuality and body changes go much easier. An example of the appropriate use of humor would be for parents to laugh as they reflect on their own experiences while growing up.

Parents can make sure that *pre-teens* receive the information they will need to make wise choices as *teens*. One of the developmental tasks of adolescence is to rebel against authority. So, it makes sense for parents to talk with their children about such matters as the need for sexual abstinence or birth control, the dangers of sexually

9—12 YEARS

transmitted diseases, and the way to make wise decisions, *before* that rebellious stage.

In addition to giving them information needed, parents of nine-through twelve-year-olds can help their children learn how to say no. In teaching children of all ages that their bodies are their own and that they don't have to let others touch them, we help prepare them to resist the peer pressure to engage in sexual intercourse before they are ready. Allow them to practice making good decisions by giving them the freedom to make choices in other areas.

Since children and youth need physical contact, one way to meet this need is to embrace our sons and daughters more frequently. In our family, no excuse is needed for hugging our children at any time. We have also found that a back-rub or foot massage is almost always appreciated by every member of our family.

Parents can encourage positive self-images. Parents of daughters can help girls feel good about being women by encouraging them to stand up for themselves. Our daughters need to know that putting themselves down, particularly in comparison to boys, is not a way to enhance femininity. It is not unfeminine to be successful, or to be a good athlete, or to be competitive. But it can injure one's self-esteem to say, "I feel like I shouldn't win, so I won't even try." If girls do this frequently in sports, a similar negative attitude may carry over into other male-female relationships. Parents can encourage their sons to welcome competition from girls, rather than to feel threatened by it. They might also discourage excessive competitiveness between male peers. Boys may need extra convincing of their worth simply because they are who they are and not because they are better than another boy.

As our children get older, it becomes less and less appropriate to say "This is the way *everyone* your age acts," "This is what *everyone* your age thinks," or "This is how *everyone* your age feels." By sixth grade, girls and boys represent a wide range of developmental levels and personal interests, making it impossible to describe the typical twelve-year-old. Moms and dads observe their children and, knowing that each is unique, encourage the development of this personal identity. Yet, it is not unusual for boys and girls to worry about being different. All persons need assurance that they are normal and will be accepted by their friends and by their society.

The openness and support of their parents can make it easier for children to be themselves. Conversely, parents can make it hard for their children when they insist upon particular behaviors or play favorites with the son or daughter who most closely reflects parental beliefs or values. Such parents often push their children into doing things so that others will think them acceptable, when it is really the parents who are worried about being accepted. An example of this is the story of Jacob and Esau, found in Genesis 25 and 27. Although Jacob and Esau were twins, their appearance, interests, and personalities were worlds apart. Esau had a red complexion, thick hair, a hearty appreciation of the open country, and the tendency to act impulsively. To Isaac, the boys' father, Esau was a man after his own heart. Jacob had a lighter, smooth complexion, preferred the quietness of staying near home, and tended to analyze a situation before taking action. Jacob was his mother Rebekah's favorite.

Rebekah was worried that Jacob would not receive the blessing and acknowledgement she felt that he deserved from his father. She insisted that Jacob pretend to have the physical characteristics and even the typical smell of a real man of the earth, thus tricking Isaac into believing that he was Esau. When Esau came home and discovered that he had been cheated, he asked the heart-rending question that all parents need to take seriously: "Do you have only one blessing, father? Bless me too, father!" (Genesis 27:38).

We need to support our children in their uniqueness and not force them into the mold of the average girl or boy. We should affirm their search to identify what masculinity and feminity means to them personally, instead of fathers saying, "If you want to be a man, you must be just like me," or mothers, "If you want to be a woman, you must be just like me."

9—12 YEARS

A Prayer for Understanding

O God, what a responsibility and privilege it is to be a parent. As the psalmist says, children are a gift from God. Help us to be worthy parents!

Enable us to appreciate the differences between boys and girls. Help us to recognize and to seize opportunities to affirm our children as sexual beings. Give us wisdom and understanding at each stage of their development so that we might be enhancers, not destroyers, of their healthy sexual identity. Amen.

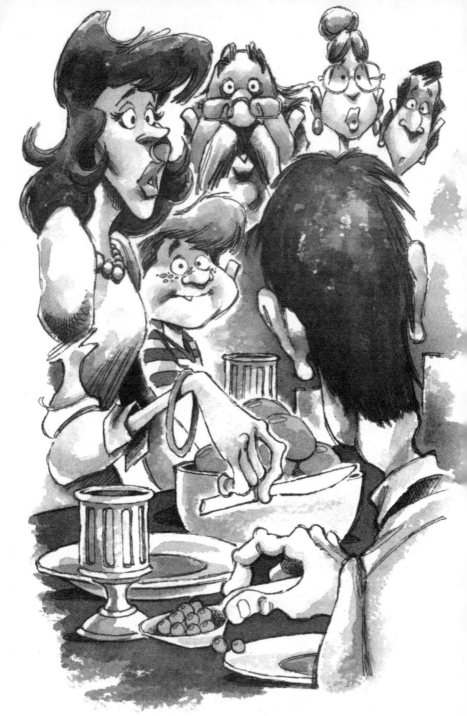

"Uh . . . we'll discuss THAT after dinner!"

CHAPTER 4

THE QUESTION BOX

PART I—QUESTIONS ABOUT SEX

How Can I Make Talks With My Children Go More Easily?

Many parents are frightened with the prospect of talking about sex. We are embarrassed and uncomfortable, concerned that our knowledge and expertise are inadequate. How could we possibly say *that* word? How can we ever explain *that* in a way that a child could understand? What if our children bring up the subject of sex during a family holiday meal or at another inappropriate time? What if we give them the wrong ideas? What if they decide to misuse the sexual information they are given?

Children can be unpredictable. We must be as prepared as possible to both respond to their questions when asked and to initiate conversations when questions *aren't* asked. There are some practical things we can do to make sexuality discussions with our children go more easily. Children will feel more secure in talking when they sense our warmth and openness. Do we demonstrate a positive attitude toward life in general and sex in particular? Do we listen carefully to our childrens' questions and take their concerns seriously? If we do, our children will come to value our discussions and will usually be glad they risked talking.

Matthew gives a beautiful picture of Jesus' openness to children. Jesus wanted the children to be with him, liked to hold them, and became irritated with people who considered them a nuisance. "Let the children come to me and do not stop them, because the Kingdom of heaven belongs to such as these" (Matthew 19:14). "Whoever welcomes in my name one such child as this, welcomes me" (Matthew 18:5). Jesus loved and respected children. We show by our words and actions that *we* love and respect our children. We can be available for them, call them to us, stand up for them, and surround them with loving, gentle arms and prayers.

Even parents who find it easy to talk about almost anything else may discover that the topic of sex throws them into a panic. Many adults have been taught that sex is a taboo subject. If this is your situation, it may help to realize that you are not obligated to tell your children about the private, personal areas of your life. You can talk about sexuality and still be discrete. Try not to let your uneasiness or nervousness be a reason to avoid talking with your child, especially when he or she asks you a question. Your child looks up to you and needs to know what you think and what you feel. Try to relax and be yourself. Take several deep breaths. If you feel embarrassed and nervous, why not admit such feelings? You might say, "I'm feeling a little uncomfortable, but I do want to talk. I'm glad that you decided to ask me."

When children come to you with questions, make sure you understand what it is they want to know. Listen carefully, and don't over-anticipate. Remember the story in which a small child asks, "Where did I come from?" The mother launches into a full-scale description of the reproductive process, then asks, "but Johnny, why did you want to know?" Johnny replies, "Well, Henry said *he* came from Kalamazoo." It is easy to give our children answers to questions they weren't even asking.

All times and settings are not condusive to conversations about sexuality. Children do not always realize that certain words are not normally discussed or used in public. You may be at a church function, with the pastor sitting on one side of your family and an elderly widow sitting on the other, when your youngster decides to ask you the meaning of a particular slang term. When this happens to us, we give a brief explanation, then firmly but kindly say, "I will tell you more about it when we get home. This is not the proper time." If proper times are provided on a regular basis, children will learn to save their questions for such moments.

We have also found that it helps to give private attention to each child's questions. We do this for several reasons. One is that Kathy and Timmy are four years apart in age. Timothy may not be interested in Kathryn's concerns or may not be able to understand the answers we give her. Girls and boys may feel embarrassed to talk about personal issues with a sibling of the opposite sex present, especially if they can't trust that other person not to giggle or tease (and brothers and sisters are notorious for both). At the same time, the advantage of such discussions is that it responds to the curiosity that boys have about girls, and girls have about boys. You will need to be sensitive to your children and their needs at this point.

In our society, fathers appear to experience more discomfort in discussing sexual issues with their children than mothers do. Recent surveys by sociologist Susan Bennett[1] indicate that American fathers assume little responsibility for their children's sex education. In general, mothers talk some with their daughters, and less with their sons. Father-daughter and father-son conversations are usually negligible. However, Bennett found that where fathers and mothers share the tasks of discipline, childcare, and household chores, there is a significantly more favorable environment for sex education. So, mothers can make sexuality talks with children go more easily by encouraging Dad to help with the diapers, dishes, and discipline, assist with homework, and tuck their sons and daughters into bed.

What Words Do You Use?

Sometimes the hardest thing in talking about sex is choosing the right words. Many parents avoid using the proper terms, simply bacause they have not had the opportunity to practice actually *saying* those terms out loud. They may mislabel acts, saying, "They are sleeping together" instead of "They are having sexual intercourse," or "Do you need to wee-wee?" instead of "Do you need to urinate?" Sometimes parents will use no specific word at all, but just say, "Don't do *that*" or "Don't touch *that*."

We can teach even our young children to use correct terms for their body parts. Explanation of slang and street language helps children to connect it with the proper terminology. Parents should not use difficult words simply for the purpose of being scientifically accurate. Accurate information may not be accurately understood, especially when a child is young. Be clear, direct, and matter-of-fact. If you use a difficult word, make certain the child knows what you are talking about. Don't give long, involved explanations. Remember that your tone of voice, facial expression, how close you sit together, and whether or not you are touching all convey a message as well.

A good answer to a question about sex is one that uses words that help children to form a solid basis of understanding. A good answer attempts to explain the feelings and emotions that accompany the process of growing up. It will have heart, not simply facts.

What About Giving My Child A Book?

Adults who feel uncomfortable talking about sex may think: "I'll give my child a book instead!" They may have the book waiting in a drawer, ready to bring out when their child asks the first question. "Here, read this," they will say, thrusting the book into the child's hands and racing for safety in another room.

Giving children books to read on their own could imply that "we don't talk about these things." Books can be a valuable tool, but should not be a substitute for parent-child discussions. Parents can use books on sexuality to bring up topics, to answer questions, or to clarify any misunderstandings. A good book should comfort and inform both you and your child about sexuality. If you feel more secure using a book, why not sit down with your child to read and discuss together? Cuddle close as you read. By your embrace, your child will be able to see that this is an inviting topic, not a frightening one.

Many excellent resources, ranging from picture books about new babies to detailed biological textbooks, are available in bookstores and in the public library. Some libraries will have these books right on the shelves; others may maintain a "by permission only" section. When choosing a book about sex for your child, look for one that gives accurate information, is appropriate for the child's age, treats sexuality with dignity, does not perpetuate myths, and does not talk down to the child. The list of recommended resources at the end of this book lists several titles which we recommend.

Created by God: About Human Sexuality for Older Girls and Boys is a companion resource to BEFORE THEY ASK (both published by Graded Press). It offers basic information about sex and human development, setting this information in the context of Christian values and positive human relationships. Children who love to read may be interested in fictional books that discuss sexuality issues. Lucille Clifton's *The Times They Used To Be* includes the subject of menstruation, and Judy Blume's *Are You There God? It's Me, Margaret* is the story of a girl's anxieties about puberty. Blume's *Then Again, Maybe I Won't* presents the problems of adolescent boys. *A Little Demonstration Of Affection*, by Elizabeth Winthrop, raises the issue of incest; and *The Longest Weekend*, by Honor Arundel, is about an unwed mother. *I'll Get There. It Better Be Worth The Trip*, by John Donovan; and *The Man Without a Face*, by Isabelle Holland, both deal with homosexuality; and Norma Klein's books, *It's Not What You*

Expect and *Mom, The Wolf Man and Me,* address the issue of extramarital affairs. If your child is reading one of these books, read along, raise questions concerning the characters' values, emotions, and behaviors, and be available to discuss your child's questions.

Fact-Giving—Does It Work?

Parents sometimes wonder if talking to their children about sexuality will do any good. Does giving our kids the facts ensure that they won't experiment with sexual intercourse before they are married? Does sex education guarantee that they will form positive relationships with persons of the opposite sex later in life or that they will make good choices concerning the use of birth control?

A survey taken in 1981 by the Alan Guttmacher Institute shows that teens who had received formal sex education training were no more likely to be sexually active than those who had not. Sex education will not cause a person to go out and experiment with sex. But students who had sex education were more likely to use contraceptives and were less likely to become pregnant. Parents may say, "But I don't want my children to use contraceptives. I don't want them having intercourse until they are married." We too share that desire for our daughter and son. We must not allow ourselves, however, to believe that children who go to church will not be interested in sex. Research informs us that students who describe themselves as having faith in God and who attend church regularly are not more likely than other students to abstain from sexual intercourse.

Fact-giving alone is not enough, but it is important. Our children will learn about sex, if not from their parents, then from their friends, music, television, and the movies. Much of the information which they learn from these other sources will be inaccurate and misleading. We must see that they receive correct information upon which to build responsible decision-making.

Parents of grade school children may be shocked to learn that the greatest risk for out-of-wedlock pregnancy occurs among adolescents who have been having sexual relationships for only a few months. Adolescents often resent adult intrusion and, once sexual activity has begun, communication might be almost impossible. Our sons and daughters need to know the facts about sex while they are still in grade school.

There is more to sexuality training than teaching biological facts or insisting that our sons and daughters "stay out of trouble". Our children need to be aware of the emotions and desires that they will have as they mature, and they will need to be able to manage them. We want our children to form positive values, to realize that sexuality is a major area of vulnerability, and to understand that sex should not be used for destructive or exploitive purposes. We want them to feel good about themselves, to be sensitive to the needs and feelings of others, and to be able to love.

How Much Information Is Too Much?

Parents should realize that they will never cover all of the important things they want to say about sex in one sitting. Sex education is not a one-session event. It is a life-time process. We have the freedom, then, to decide that "this is enough information for now." If we are discussing a question with our child and he or she begins to fidget and lose interest, it is probably time to go on to something else. Young children do not have a long attention span and may not be able to concentrate on a lengthy explanation.

Remember that there are stages in the development of children's understanding of sex and birth. Babies do not think in the same way that five-year-olds do. If we give children information that is geared to a higher level of understanding, they may not be able to put the facts all together. Too many details will be confusing and may make young children feel stupid, ashamed, or fearful.

If your child becomes terribly embarrassed or upset during a discussion, change to a less-threatening topic and return to your talk at another time. Ask questions to find out what the child is thinking before you attempt to give any more information.

We have a list of "Don'ts" which we feel are important for parents to remember when talking with children about sex. Don't use sex to frighten your children, such as the old masturbation myths of blindness or sterility. Don't start by telling fables such as "the stork brought you" or untruths. Don't tease your child about sexuality. Don't punish your child if he engages in sex play or asks embarrassing questions. And don't be emotionally dishonest yourself—examine your attitudes and feelings and accept the range of emotions that you might feel.

What If My Child Never Asks Questions?

Some parents worry about the answers that they should give to their children's questions. Other parents worry because their children never seem to have any questions to be answered. What should parents do if their children never ask questions about sex?

We do not have to wait for our children to bring up the subject. We can use the opportunities of everyday life to talk about sexual issues. People sometimes call these opportunities *teachable moments*. They are the innumerable small situations that might occur at any time—moments which we can use as springboards for sharing our thoughts and values. Talk about Aunt Carolyn's new baby. Stop at the window of the pet shop to admire the new puppies. Look at the lingerie section in the Sear's catalog. Discuss the evening news. Comment on how tall your children are growing or how mature they appear to be. Watch TV with your children and ask them what they think or how they feel about some of the "sexy" scenes. The possibilities are endless. The trick for parents is learning how to recognize and take advantage of these opportunities.

In our family, we have found that the perfect time to talk about sex is not programmed. Our most productive discussions occur while driving in the car, while eating an after-school snack, while taking a bath, or when it is time to go to sleep. We have never specifically set aside a time to talk about sex. But we do ask our children questions such as, "How do the boys in your class feel about the girls?" "How do you think mommies get to be mommies?" "Do you want to be a daddy when you grow up?" A child's unexpected entrance when we are using the bathroom or changing clothes can be used to talk about the adult body. We include our children in adult discussions of the news, so that in talking about surrogate mothers, homosexuality, or child abuse, we can listen to our children's feelings and worries as well as help them to learn about human sexuality.

PART II—QUESTIONS AND SAMPLE RESPONSES

No two children are exactly alike—each has a unique set of interests, questions, and worries. No two parents are alike, either. Parents all have their own styles of responding to children—styles that build on their personal sets of values and experiences. There is no one correct way to talk with a child about sexuality. But it can sometimes be informative to "eavesdrop" on the conversations of other parents and children, if only to discover the variety of questions and possible responses that exist. On the following pages, you will find a series of questions that children at different age levels might ask and a short response which might be offered. These are not intended to be the only or even the best possible responses. But we hope they will encourage you to think ahead about the answers you may someday want to give to your children.

As you read some of the responses, you may find them too complicated. Children will probably not be able to understand all of this information, especially the first time they hear it. Children are often curious about topics that are difficult to explain in simple terms. You may want to simplify the language, or use fewer details. Be prepared to have your child ask you the same question several times. Do not underestimate your child, however. He or she may be able to grasp much more than you realize.

Questions Preschool Children Might Ask

Young children, fascinated with babies, might wonder—

Where was I kept before you married Daddy?
You weren't kept anywhere because you didn't exist yet. To make a baby, you need a man and woman to be the baby's father and mother. A new baby is created from an ovum inside the mother and a sperm from the father.

How does the baby get inside the mother?
The mother's body makes an ovum. The father's body makes a sperm which he places into the mother's body with his penis. When the ovum and the sperm cell join together, a baby starts to grow.

Do unmarried people ever have babies?
Yes, sometimes they do. You don't have to be married to have a baby, but it does take both a man and a woman in order for the baby to be formed.

Can a man be pregnant with a baby?
No, men's bodies are different from women's bodies. Mothers have a special place, called the uterus, for the baby. Mothers also have a special passage inside their bodies, called the vagina, where the baby comes out when it is ready. Men and boys do not have a uterus or vagina.

Can a baby cry before it is born?

No, an unborn baby doesn't cry. In order to make the sound of crying, you have to have air in your lungs. This air moves up into your voice box to make the crying sound. But a baby doesn't use its lungs for breathing until after it is born, so it can't cry.

Does the baby come out through the belly button?

No, a baby comes out of the mother through her vagina, which is between her legs.

Where does the milk come from when you nurse the baby?

The mother's body makes the milk for her baby. The milk is formed by special glands in her breasts.

Tucking a pillow under her shirt and pretending to be pregnant, a child announces, "I want to have my own baby now. Why can't I?"

Your body isn't ready to have babies. As you grow older, your body will change so that you could have a baby if you chose to.

Daddy, I'm going to marry you when I grow up!

You must think I'm somebody special to want to marry me. Thank you! Lots of boys and girls think about the same thing. But you can't marry me because I am your father. When you grow up, you can fall in love with a man and get married to him. If you have children, he will be their father and I will be their grandfather!

Preschool children have questions about their bodies and about differences between boys and girls. They may want to know—

Why don't girls have a penis?

Girls' bodies are different from boys. They have a vulva, which is the part of a girl's body that is between her legs.

Why are boy's bathrooms different from girl's bathrooms?

When you urinate, the fluid comes out of the urethra. A girl's urethra is inside her body, so it is easier for her to urinate while sitting. A boy's urethra is in his penis, and he can urinate standing up. This is why boy's and girl's bathrooms are different—boy's bathrooms often have urinals to use while standing, and girl's bathrooms do not.

Daddy has a scratchy beard. Why doesn't Mommy?

When men and boys grow up, hair grows on their faces. Women don't have lots of hair on their faces.

What is the belly button for?

When you eat, the food inside of you becomes broken up into very, very small bits. Your blood then carries the food to the parts of your body. When you breathe, your blood carries oxygen from the air to all the parts of your body. When a woman is pregnant, she shares her food and oxygen with her baby. It gets from the mother to the baby through the umbilical cord. After babies are born, they don't need the umbilical cord any more. It is tied and cut near your tummy, and it leaves this indention called the navel or belly button. The navel doesn't do anything now—it just marks the spot where you were once connected to your mother.

Questions Younger Elementary Children Might Ask

Younger grade school children have many questions about the human body, such as:

Why do grownups have so much hair on their bodies?

When a person's body becomes mature or grown up, it produces chemicals called hormones. Hormones cause hair to grow. Both men and women have hair under their arms, on their legs, and in their genital area (around the sex organs). Men also have hair on their faces and often on their chests.

Why do women menstruate? What is a period?

Menstruation, commonly called a period, is one part of the reproductive cycle—which means it is part of the way a woman's body gets ready to have a baby. About once a month, an ovum is released by the ovaries. The uterus begins to build up a rich lining of blood and tissue which will serve as a bed to help the ovum grow. Most of the time, the ovum is not fertilized by a sperm cell. Since there is no baby in the uterus, this lining is not needed. Menstruation is when the blood and tissue from the uterus flow out of the body.

What are the testicles for?

The testicles are the male glands that produce the sperm cells. The testicles also produce the male sex hormones that cause body changes such as the growth of the penis, the appearance of pubic hair, and a lowered voice.

What is circumcision?

The skin on the penis of a newborn baby boy covers the end of his penis. This skin is sometimes removed in an operation called circumcision. The operation is usually done shortly after he is born. Some boys are not circumcised. Circumcised and uncircumcised penises look different, but they work just the same.

Grade school children may wonder about terms which are unfamiliar to them, especially if they hear these words used in movies or TV or by their friends—

What is a virgin? Can a boy be a virgin?

A virgin is someone who has not had sexual intercourse. Both boys and girls can be virgins.

What is a prostitute?

A prostitute is someone who is paid for taking part in a sexual act.

What is a homosexual?

Homosexuals are persons who are sexually attracted to or sexually active with other persons of the same sex. Women homosexuals are called *lesbians*; male homosexuals are often referred to as *gay*.

Younger elementary children are often curious about the act of sexual intercourse—

Why do people have sex? Why would they want to?

Sexual intercourse is a way that two people can demonstrate their love for one another. It can provide great physical pleasure and closeness and is also the way to have children .

What happens during sexual intercourse?

Before a man and woman have sexual intercourse, the man's penis becomes larger and more firm. This is called an erection. The woman's vagina becomes wet and relaxed. Intercourse takes place when the man pushes his penis into the woman's vagina, and they move their bodies together. The man usually experiences an ejaculation, where a fluid, called semen (which contains sperm) is squirted from his penis. If a sperm cell joins with an ovum in the woman's body, a baby begins. A baby does not begin, however, every time they have intercourse.

What is birth control?

Birth control means choosing whether or when to have a baby.

Grade school children are still very interested in babies and in pregnancy—

How does a cell turn into a baby?

When the ovum joins with a sperm cell, it is fertilized. The fertilized ovum then begins the process of cell division. The cell divides into two cells. Then each of those cells divides into two, and so on. Some of the cells will eventually develop into fingers, toes, and all of the rest of the baby's body.

What causes twins?

When one fertilized ovum divides into two completely separate cells, twins will develop. These twins will look almost exactly alike, so they are called identical twins. There is also another way that twins are formed. Sometimes two separate ova (more than one ovum) join with two different sperm and then each of them begins to develop into a new human being. These twins will not look exactly the same, but differ just like regular brothers and sisters differ from each other. We call them fraternal twins.

Why does a baby look like its parents?

The ovum, which comes from the baby's mother, and the sperm, which come from the father, both contain chromosomes with genes. The genes carry "messages" to the newly formed child. The combination of genes that you receive from your parents determines what you will look like. You will be like one parent in some ways and like the other parent in other ways. You will also have features that are blends of both.

What decides a baby's sex?

The sex chromosomes do. The sex chromosome that carries instructions for being male is called a Y chromosome, and the sex chromosome that carries instructions for being female is called an X chromosome. If a baby has two X chromosomes, it is a girl. But if a baby has a combination of an X and a Y chromosome, it is a boy.

How can you tell if a baby is going to be a girl or a boy?

Most parents do not know whether their child is a boy or girl until the moment the baby is born. However, doctors can use sound vibrations (called ultrasound) to look at the baby before it is born, and the ultrasound pictures often show the doctor and the parents what the baby's sex is.

How long does it take for a baby to be formed?

It takes about 280 days (9 months) for a baby to develop.

How does a woman know she is going to have a baby?

A woman can often guess that she is going to have a baby when she misses a menstrual period, and if she feel nauseous (called having morning sickness). The doctor can test the woman's urine to see if it shows traces of hormones from the baby.

Can a baby hear before it is born?

Yes, the unborn baby can probably hear voices, the beat of the mother's heart, and the noise of music and traffic outside.

How does a baby breathe inside the mother?

The umbilical cord carries oxygen to the baby from the placenta.

How does a baby "go to the bathroom" before he is born?

The umbilical cord carries wastes away from the baby.

How is a baby actually born?

The mother's vagina expands, and as muscles contract or suddenly get shorter, they begin to push the baby out. These contractions are called labor. The baby comes down through the mother's cervix (the opening of the uterus), usually head-first.

How long does labor usually take?

It depends. First babies usually take longer to be born. Labor may take as long as 10 to 16 hours or more.

Does labor hurt?

Yes, labor contractions are painful for mothers. Some parents take childbirth classes to help them learn to control the pain through breathing. Others may use medication to control the pain.

Does the baby ever get stuck?

The labor contractions cause the cervix to open wide enough to allow the baby to pass through. If there is a danger that the baby will have difficulty passing through the birth canal, the doctor may perform an operation called a caesarean section to deliver the baby through the abdomen.

Does cutting the umbilical cord hurt the baby?

No, the umbilical cord has no nerve endings in it, so cutting the cord does not hurt.

What is a miscarriage?

A miscarriage is when a baby is born before it has developed enough to live outside the mother's body. It usually occurs when something has happened to interfere with the fetus' normal growth.

Questions Older Grade School Students Might Ask

Boys and girls have questions about the changes their bodies are (or will soon be) experiencing.

What is the male reproductive system like?

Sperm cells are produced in the testicles, which are held in the scrotum. The scrotum helps to keep the sperm cells at the correct temperature. When it is cold, a small muscle in the scrotum pulls the testicles up close to the body for warmth.

The sperm cells mature as they move through the epididymis—a series of tiny tubes attached to the back of each testicle. They then move through tubes called vas deferens, where they are mixed with fluids called semen. The sperm and semen move into the male urethra, a tube in the center of the penis.

When semen is to leave the body, the penis tissue fills with blood, causing the penis to become larger, firmer, and to stand out from the body. This is called an erection. Semen can then be forcefully ejected from the body by contractions of the prostate gland and the seminal vesicles. This is called an ejaculation.

Does an ejaculation happen with every erection?

No. The penis can become erect for reasons besides sexual stimulation, such as when lifting a heavy load, wearing clothing that is tight, having to urinate, or even for no apparent reason at all. These erections usually go away after a few minutes.

Why do boys have "wet dreams"?

As a boy's body begins to physically mature, it constantly produces sperm. The sperm accumulates in the tubes leading from the testes. When excess sperm has accumulated, the body gets rid of it by an ejaculation of semen, often during sleep. This ejaculation is called a nocturnal emission or wet dream. It may or may not be accompanied by sex-related dreams.

Is semen the same as urine?

No. Urine is a yellowish liquid body waste that is formed in the kidneys and stored in the bladder. Semen is a thick, whitish fluid that carries sperm cells from the testicles. Both urine and semen leave the body through the urethra, but never at the same time.

Is it normal for one testicle to be bigger or to hang lower in the scrotum than the other?

Yes, one testicle—usually the left one—normally hangs lower than the other. This is a way that the body has to protect the testicles from being painfully pressed together. If one or both of the testicles has not descended into the scrotum, a doctor should correct the situation.

Does the size of the penis make a difference?

Boys and men often worry about how tall they are, how muscular they are, how much hair they have on their bodies, and about the size of their genitals. They compare themselves to other boys and men and, if they are smaller or have less hair, may begin feeling bad about themselves. The size of the penis is not related to sexual capability, but it can be related to how one feels about his body. It's something you don't have any control over, so it is best to accept your body as it is. These feelings are very common. No one your age wants to feel different. You're not alone.

What is the female reproductive system like?

A woman has two ovaries, each about the size of a pecan, in the lower part of her abdomen. The ovaries hold the ovum or ova. About once a month, one of the ovaries will release an ovum—this is called ovulation. The ovum enters the fallopian tubes, where it may be fertilized by a sperm cell from a male. The fallopian tubes lead to the uterus, a hollow organ about three inches long. If an ovum is fertilized, it implants itself onto the wall of the uterus and grows there, with the uterus stretching to make room for the fetus. The lower part of the uterus is the cervix. It connects to the vagina, which leads to the outside of the body. When babies are born, they are generally delivered through the vagina.

When will I begin to menstruate?

A girl usually begins to menstruate sometime between the ages of 10 and 14. Some girls begin before this, and others may be 16 or 17 before they first menstruate. Menstruation is a sign that you are capable of reproduction.

How do you know when you are about to have your period?

Many girls find that they feel "puffy" or bloated a few days before their period begins because their bodies retain an extra amount of water. This water can even cause a several-pound weight gain. Some girls may feel irritable, tense, or depressed during this time. Others experience backaches or slight pain in the uterine area or may find that their breasts are very sensitive to touch.

What is this white stuff that gets on my panties?

A woman's body secretes a white fluid called a vaginal discharge, especially right before the menstrual period or around the time of ovulation. This fluid is caused by bacteria in the vagina which provide natural protection against germs and infections. This is normal. However, if the discharge has an unpleasant odor or causes burning or itching, it is usually caused by an infection and should be treated by a doctor.

Sometimes I "touch myself." Does this mean I am strange or doing something wrong?

No. Obtaining physical pleasure by touching or rubbing our sex organs is called masturbation. It is normal and not harmful unless we become overly preoccupied with it. This is one of the ways that we discover more about our bodies.

Older grade school youth have questions about pregnancy and sexual intercourse.

How many times does it take to "do it" before you get pregnant? Can a girl become pregnant the first time?

It only takes one act of sexual intercourse to become pregnant. One does not become pregnant every time she has intercourse.

Is there a certain time when a woman can get pregnant?

A woman is most likely to become pregnant at the time of ovulation (when the ovum is released), and on the days immediately before and after. This occurs approximately 14 days after the beginning of the menstrual cycle.

If you miss your period, does that mean that you are pregnant?

It might, if you have had sexual intercourse. However, stress, illness, losing a large amount of weight, or participation in strenuous exercise can cause a period to be late or missed.

Can you have a baby when you are 10 years old?

The beginning of menstruation is a sign that your body is physically capable of pregnancy. Some 10-year-olds have already reached puberty, and it would be possible for them to have a baby.

Can a girl become pregnant without intercourse?

Usually not. While it is unlikely, pregnancy is possible if semen is ejaculated near the vaginal opening. The semen may seep in without penetration of the penis inside the woman's body. In addition, if a man has semen on his hands when he touches a woman's vagina, the sperm may enter her body in this way.

What kinds of birth control methods are there?

There are many different methods of birth control. The only 100 percent effective method is not to have sexual intercourse. This is called abstinence. Some women take birth control pills, which contain artificial hormones which stop the release of ova. Other women use an intrauterine device (IUD) made of metal or plastic which a doctor inserts into the uterus. Some women block sperm from entering the uterus by using a diaphragm—a rubber cap that fits over the cervix, or by placing sperm-killing creams or foams into the vagina. A man can wear a condom on his penis during sexual intercourse. A condom is like a large, rolled-up balloon that is unrolled over the penis to catch the sperm. Some couples use Natural Family Planning, which requires couples to watch for signs of ovulation and then to refrain from sexual intercourse on those days when conception is possible. Because of the difficulty of determining exactly when ovulation occurs, this method can be unreliable.

Surgical methods of birth control are called sterilization. A man might have a vasectomy, in which the vas deferens are cut and tied; a woman might have a tubal ligation in which her fallopian tubes are cut and tied.

What happens in an abortion?

Abortion is the act of stopping a pregnancy. One method is dilation and curettage (D & C), in which the lining of the uterus is scraped to disconnect the embryo from the uterine wall. Another method is vacuum aspiration, which uses suction to pull the lining and the embryo from the uterine wall.

Does it hurt to "do it" with a boy?

Sexual intercourse is generally pleasurable for women and men. As a couple leads up to sexual intercourse, their bodies prepare. Men are ready for intercourse before their partners are ready, and must be patient. If a woman is rushed, intercourse can be painful. The first few experiences of intercourse can be uncomfortable for both the woman and the man—generally due to their nervousness and their inability to relax.

What is rape?

Rape means being forced to have sexual intercourse against your will. It is against the law. Rape by someone with whom you are on a date is referred to as date rape and is also against the law.

What is incest?

Incest is having sexual relations with a blood relative. It is illegal in the United States and forbidden in most parts of the world.

What is STD?

STD stands for Sexually Transmitted Diseases—diseases passed through sexual contact. If not treated, these diseases can cause mental illness, crippling, damage to the heart and other parts of the body, or even death. Common STD's include gonorrhea, syphilis, herpes, trichominiasis, and chlamydia.

What is AIDS?

AIDS is the abbreviation for Acquired Immune Deficiency Syndrome, a disease which causes a breakdown of the body's system for fighting off disease. AIDS is transmitted through the exchange of body fluids. This takes place during heterosexual and homosexual intercourse, through the sharing of contaminated needles by drug users, and from an infected mother to her unborn baby. Some present AIDS victims were infected when they received contaminated blood during a transfusion. Because of improved blood testing procedures, this is no longer possible.

How can a person keep from getting AIDS?

The best way to avoid contracting AIDS is not to have sexual intercourse. Persons who do engage in sexual intercourse should use condoms for protection. Because AIDS is also spread by contaminated needles, you should not use drugs and should never share hypodermic needles.

Can both men and women carry sexually transmitted diseases?

Yes, both sexes can contract and carry these diseases. A pregnant woman can also pass the disease to her unborn baby.

Boys and girls in the upper grade school years may be beginning to have questions and worries about relationships and emotions.

What makes me feel so moody?

As you grow, your view of the world changes. You become more aware of what is going on around you. Your family once seemed secure and satisfying and demanded very little from you. But now that you are older, you have greater responsibilities, more concerns about the future, and increased personal insecurity. These can all make you feel moody. In addition, your hormones are causing your body to develop, and these hormonal changes can often cause mood swings.

What should I do when someone teases me about my body?

It hurts when someone teases you about being too big or too small or makes fun of the changes your body is going through. Remember that change is normal and good and that everyone develops at his or her own rate. The persons doing the teasing are probably unsure of or frightened by some of their own body changes. If an adult teases you, it may be because he or she is not emotionally ready to see you grow up. Try to be understanding, have a good sense of humor, and don't let the teasing damage your positive self-image.

Sometimes I daydream about sexy things. Is there something wrong with me? Does this mean I'm perverted?

Many people have sexual fantasies. Sometimes people have sexual urges and desires, but they know that acting on those urges would be inappropriate, so they experience them in their imagination instead. This can be healthy and helpful. But sometimes people get caught up in their fantasies and are unable to think about anything else. Or they may lose sight of the difference between what is real and what is imaginary and may try to live out their fantasies, hurting themselves and others in the process.

Do many people have sex before marriage? What happens if they do?

While many persons do have sex before marriage, the numbers do not make it right. Such persons risk emotional hurt, pregnancy, disease, and often destroy the relationship they thought they would fulfill with intercourse.

How can people control their desire for sex?

People can learn to control their sexual emotions in the same way that they control their other emotions. Toddlers have to learn to control their temper tantrums. Kindergarten children must conquer their fear of going to school. We must discover how to set limits and standards for ourselves, then we must learn to live within those limits. Another way to control our desire for sex is not to allow ourselves to think mainly or exclusively about sex. We can exercise, keep busy, and have other interests, goals, and activities in addition to our interest in sex.

How can you say "No?"

If someone wants you to have a sexual relationship that you are not ready for or just do not want to have, you have the right to simply say, "No, I don't want to." You do not have to explain or apologize. Remember that the consequences of sexual activity can be long-lasting and life-changing. Be sure that you are ready for those possibilities before you say "Yes."

Is it ever okay to have sex?

When two people care deeply for each other and have made a commitment to each other, sexual intercourse can be a beautiful expression of their love. It is a way in which a husband and wife can give one another the gift of pleasure and intimacy. It is also the way in which a couple can take part in the creation of a new life.

I think having a baby would be fun! What could be so bad about having a baby when you're my age?

Having a baby is an adult thing to do. It's understandable for young people to want to do adult things. But, while babies are cute and precious, they are also tremendous responsibilities—not toys. They need constant care. It takes thousands of dollars to pay for the food, diapers, and health care they need. When someone as young as you has a child, it is almost always impossible for the mother to earn enough money to provide for the baby's needs. If you had a baby, you would have to grow up very fast and would probably feel cheated out of your own childhood. Also, when the mother is very young, her baby's health can be put in danger—the baby has a much greater chance of being born too early or of having a low birth-weight.

Why do our bodies begin to change and mature so long before we are ready to get married and raise a family?

Years ago, people got married at a much younger age. It didn't take years of educational training to prepare them for their life's work, so they often had the means of providing for a family when they were still very young. It was usually helpful for a family to have a large number of children, so a couple would start early to build that family. But today, while such factors as better nutrition and health care cause our bodies to mature even earlier than they used to, it takes longer and longer to become prepared to live and work in society as an adult. As a result, the waiting period between the time our bodies are ready for sexual intercourse and the time we are mature enough in other ways seems so long.

Older elementary children have worries about homosexuality and unusual sexual activities or preferences.

If you have a crush on someone of your own sex, does that make you a homosexual?

No, a homosexual is someone who remains sexually attracted only to a person or persons of his or her own sex. One crush or one experience does not make a person a homosexual.

What does AC/DC mean?

AC/DC is a slang term for bisexuality. A bisexual is a person who is sexually attracted to or sexually active with both women and men. The term AC/DC comes from the two different types of electrical current—alternating and direct.

What is a transexual?

Transexuals are persons who believe themselves to be one sex mentally and emotionally, while they are the opposite sex physically. Some of these persons undergo sex-change operations to make them more like the sex that they *feel* they are.

What is artificial insemination?

Artificial insemination means placing sperm into a woman's vagina by means of a syringe. Doctors may perform artificial insemination when a couple has not been able to conceive a child through sexual intercourse.

What is a surrogate mother?

When a couple wishes to have a baby but the woman is unable to conceive, they may arrange to have another woman become impregnated with the husband's sperm by artificial insemination. This substitute mother will carry the fetus in her body until its birth. After the child is delivered, he or she is raised by the biological father and his wife.

A Time For Silence

No matter how earnestly we wish to give our children the benefit of our knowledge, especially when they come to us with questions, we need to remember that parenthood does not give us the license to bombard our sons and daughters with talk. Our role is to be parents, not lecturers. The advice we give to our families is vitally important, but so are the moments of listening. Are we hearing what our children are saying beneath their questions? Do we understand their worries and fears? Can we tell when they are confused or embarrassed? Are we willing to admit when we don't know an answer? Do we assure our kids that *we* sometimes have questions and worries and that we understand what it means to feel embarrassed and confused? As Ecclesiastes 11:5 says, we are not experts on life.

> God made everything, and you can no
> more understand what he does than
> you understand how new life begins
> in the womb of a pregnant woman.

When our kids ask questions about what it means to be "all grown up," we should be humble! An appropriate response might be, "I don't know. I'm still growing—not my body, but my mind and my relationships." We don't need to feel that we must have an answer for every issue. Sometimes it is all right to be silent. And when we do talk, we should always try to be loving and wise.

In giving answers to our children, what we say is equaled in importance by how we say it. Answers can be a way to criticize our children, to scold or scare them, to make them feel guilty, or to place authoritative demands on them. On the other hand, our answers can be a way to nurture our families. Words can be affirming, supportive, and positive. They can enhance our children's self-esteem and build their feelings of value and worth, as well as give them the information they need about sex. As Paul says in Ephesians 4:29:

> Do not use harmful words, but only
> helpful words, the kind that build
> up and provide what is needed, so
> that what you say will do good to
> those who hear you.

If this is how we, as parents, choose our words, we can then dare to show our children Proverbs 4. This proverb, which insists that children should listen to what their parents say, is based on the assumption that parents have wisdom. It claims that parental insight brings protection, safety, and love; that knowing the right way to live gives positive direction for decision-making; that education is important to life itself; and that understanding can influence what happens in our life, even affecting our thoughts and our health.

> Children, listen to what your parents teach you.
> Pay attention, and you will have understanding.
> What I am teaching you is good, so remember it
> all. Get wisdom and insight! Do not forget or
> ignore what I say. Do not abandon wisdom, and
> she will keep you safe. Getting wisdom is the
> most important thing you can do. Listen to me,
> child. Take seriously what I am telling you, and
> you will live a long life. I have taught you wisdom
> and the right way to live. Nothing will stand in
> your way if you walk wisely, and you will not
> stumble when you run. Always remember what
> you have learned. Your education is your life—
> guard it well. Child, pay attention to what I say.
> Listen to my words. Never let them get away from
> you. Remember them and keep them in your
> heart. They will give life and health to anyone
> who understands them. Be careful how you think;
> your life is shaped by your thoughts. Look straight
> ahead with honest confidence; don't hang your
> head in shame. Plan carefully what you do, and
> whatever you do will turn out right. Avoid evil
> and walk straight ahead. Don't go one step off the
> right way.
> Proverbs 4:1–2,5–7,10–13,20–23,25–27 (adapted)

These verses can be marvelous guidelines for parents who are answering questions about sex! Do our answers give children the security and love they need to feel protected and affirmed? Will our answers help our sons and daughters make their own decisions? Are we showing our children that they don't need to be afraid of knowledge about sex, because information and understanding can make us stronger, happier, and healthier? If we can honestly answer "Yes" to these guidelines, we can "look straight ahead with honest confidence" as we communicate with our children about the important things in life.

A Prayer For Wisdom

Loving God, be near me as I talk with my children about our sexuality. Help me relate to them with trust, love, and respect. Show me how to be warm and open in my attitudes as well as my answers.

Help me listen to my child. Grant me the courage to admit my lack of knowledge when confronted with something I don't know and help me not to be afraid of my own discomfort or embarrassment. Keep me alert to recognize teachable moments and give me wisdom as I choose my words. Amen.

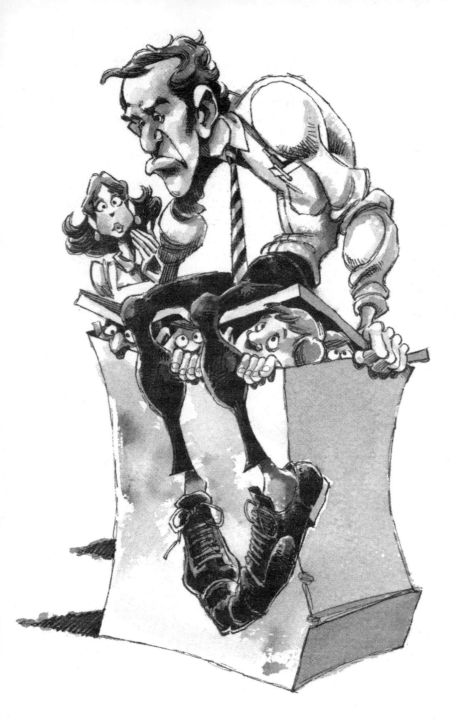

"But, Dear, you'll *have* to let them out to go to school!"

CHAPTER 5

THE REAL WORLD

Boys and Girls in a Box

When we parents take an honest look at the world in which we and our children live, we realize that sexual security is not part of the environment. In many ways, sexuality spells danger for our sons and daughters—danger found in the violence of sexual abuse and rape, the threat of AIDS and other sexually transmitted diseases, the pressure from the media to conform with its image of masculinity and femininity, the aggressive use of off-color jokes and sex-related slang terms, the lure of early sexual activity, the possibility of unwanted pregnancies, and general family stress.

As parents we may want to gather up our children, place them in a protective box, and sit on the lid until we are sure it is safe for them to emerge into the world! We can't do that, of course. Though we want to protect our children from potential dangers, we do not have the option of isolating them. They have to live in a real world complete with real dangers.

How can we, living in a society where people are hurt every day by sex, help our children to face life with a positive attitude? How can we show them that sexuality is a good gift, not a harmful one? The best protection is to be informed. Naivete, ignorance, and fear can trip us up and plunge us headfirst into sexual pitfalls. Aware of the dangers that exist, we can intentionally work against them.

Sexual Abuse of Children

Some of the most startling and troubling statistics of American society show the frequency with which children are being sexually abused. Research data accumulated by the American Humane Association in twenty-eight states reported 132,000 *confirmed* cases of child abuse in 1986. Many other cases are suspected, but have not been verified. Research suggests that one-fourth of all girls and one-sixth of all boys will be the victims of sexual abuse before they are 18 years old. Of the confirmed cases, 42 percent of the abuse was committed by parents, and 22.8 percent was committed by other relatives. Many of the other offenders were persons the child knew—a family friend, baby sitter, or neighbor. The average age of a sexually abused child is nine years old. 22.8 percent of the victims are boys.

Most cases of child molesting and incest occur at night in the home of the offender or victim—not in cars, abandoned buildings, parks, or on the schoolground. Nine out of ten offenders are men, typically under age 31.[1]

Because assailants usually warn their victims not to tell, children who are sexually assaulted are often afraid to report the incident. They worry that they will be punished, blamed, or not believed. Indeed, many parents *do* blame or punish the child who has been molested. Though they remain silent, sexually abused children may tell in other ways. They may become depressed and withdrawn or may pinch or bite themselves to inflict self-pain. They may mimic the actions of sexual intercourse during their play. Abused children may also appear to be in a daze or want to sleep for extended periods of time. They may regress in behavior, reverting to bedwetting, thumb sucking, or fearing the dark. School-aged children may do poorly in school, have frequent nightmares, or begin to act out sexually with their toys or pets. Teens who have been sexually abused may become highly emotional and experience intense fears of sexual activity. Others go to the opposite extreme and become deliberately provocative, behaving in ways that make them vulnerable to further sexual attacks. Some run away from home, become suicidal, or turn to drug and alcohol abuse.

The sexual abuse of children is not limited to any type of family or geographical location—it occurs in all racial and ethnic groups and across all economic and social levels. However, certain similarities are frequently evident. Sexually abused children and their families often appear to be socially isolated and have difficulty forming relationships outside the home. Parents in such families are often very strict, set rigid rules for relationships, and appear highly religious. Many have lived in a given community less than two years. Children in such families may be expected to assume unreasonable levels of responsibility.[2]

Children suffering from parental abuse may defend the abusive parent. They may worry that exposing the abuse would destroy family unity and happiness. When such children do seek help, they often find themselves isolated, especially if other family members (including the non-abusive parent) continue to support the offender by refusing to believe that the assault occurred.

It is characteristic for sexual abusers to deny or rationalize their actions. They may state that fondling a child's genitals is simply a way of expressing parental affection or a means for teaching the child about sex. Many parents who sexually abuse their children were themselves abused as children and may experience difficulty in coming to grips with those past experiences.

Helping Protect Your Child Against Sexual Abuse

Some parents worry that a discussion of sexual abuse will frighten their child. They decide to keep quiet about the topic, hoping they will never need to face the issue. A study conducted in Boston in 1984 found that parents from every social sector and ethnic group were uncomfortable dealing with the possibility of sexual abuse and were doing little to educate their children about it.

Helping our children to be sexually safe is just as important as teaching them the basics of fire or traffic safety. Although very young boys and girls are the most easily victimized, they can be taught to protect themselves against sexual abuse. We can teach them that their bodies are good, that their bodies belong to them, and that no one has a right to touch any part of their bodies that they do not want to be touched. We can tell them that learning to take care of and protect our bodies is a natural part of growing up and that almost every adult wants to help them be safe. Stress to your children the importance of telling someone right away if they have been abused, even if the offender threatens them into secrecy.

There are several books on the market designed to teach children about preventing sexual abuse. One is *Good Hugs and Bad Hugs—How Can You Tell?* by Angela R. Carl. This Christian activity book helps children to distinguish between good touches and unwanted ones. It teaches safety skills and assures the child of God's love no matter what has happened. Another excellent resource is *Red Flag, Green Flag People*, by J. Williams. This story and coloring book teaches children to be alert to possible dangers and to know what "red flags" to watch out for. Other resources, such as puppet plays and skits, have been developed for use in schools and day care centers. Most are designed to educate the boys and girls in a lighthearted, entertaining, and non-threatening manner, and have been used with excellent results. Encourage your school or church to investigate the use of such programs for their students.

Helping a Child Who Has Been Sexually Abused

What should you do if your child tells you that he or she has been sexually abused? First, believe the child and take the complaint seriously. Children do not usually lie about being molested. Second, assure the child that the episode is all right to talk about and was not something for which he or she is to blame. Children in such situations need to know that they are believed and that you will do everything possible to make sure the abuse stops. Focus on the emotions and needs of the child, not on the anger you feel towards the assailant. Do your best to make the child feel secure and to help him or her maintain a positive self-image.

A sexually abused child needs to receive immediate medical attention, given the possibility of physical damage and the great risk of contracting a sexually transmitted disease. Realize that the medical exam itself may be traumatic for the child and try to see that he or she feels safe and understands what is happening. If possible, use a doctor your child already knows and with whom he or she feels comfortable.

The law requires that you report suspected cases of child abuse. Contact the Human Services or Sexual Abuse Unit of your local police department, County Social Services, or call the National Abuse Hotline: 1-800-422-4453 (1-800-4A CHILD).

Rape and Incest: The Bible Touches a Sad Truth

Sexual violence is not just a modern phenomenon. Numerous Bible stories attest to the sad truth that rape and incest have been with us for thousands of years. Bible stories often depict a lust which escalates into an act of hostile violence. In 2 Samuel 13 and 14, David's son Amnon was tormented with desire for his beautiful sister, Tamar. Urged on by his friend Jonadab, Amnon planned the rape of his sister—an act viewed as an offense against the entire family. David was angry, as was Tamar's other brother, Absalom. After two years of letting his hatred for Amnon fester and grow, Absalom finally had his brother murdered in retaliation for the rape. Absalom then fled for his own life, and for years the family's unity and happiness was destroyed.

In Genesis 34, a woman named Dinah was seized and raped by a Gentile prince. His act embittered the members of the Hebrew tribe, who initiated their revenge by saying to the Gentiles, "If you want to have a relationship with one of our girls, you'll have to be circumcised." The prince's men agreed to be circumcised. While the Gentiles were recuperating, the Hebrews made a surprise attack, killed the entire tribe, and took all of the women captive. The Hebrews believed that the rape justified this retaliation.

Today, people are still subject to sexual violence, and society continues to have difficulty dealing with the problem. Considered the most serious sexual offense covered by the criminal law, rape is one of the crimes that frequently carries the death penalty. Yet in many instances, people convicted of rape do not receive stiff penalties. In California, for example, men convicted of forceable rape spend an average of only 36 months in prison—less than the average prison term for people convicted of lesser crimes. An overburdened legal system, overcrowding in prisons, and the difficulty in making convictions when the victim is the only witness are three of the factors that may explain this inequity in punishments. However, we may also need to give thought to our society's attitudes toward women and sex in general and toward rape in particular—attitudes that may contribute to such inequity.

Psychologists and sociologists have begun to categorize rapes. Separate categories exist for rape by strangers, rape by acquaintances, rape by physical violence or the threat of violence, rape based on position of authority, rape by seduction of children too young to be responsible for their actions, gang rapes, and rape during a date. While different types of rape may cause different emotions in the victims and may be viewed in different ways by society, they are all violent acts of sex committed against the will of the victim.

Date rape is one category of rape that is often difficult to prove, but like all other categories, it is illegal. Our sons and daughters need to be aware of the threat of date rape. We must teach our youth to act responsibly when dating and must stress to them that the dating relationship does not give one person the right to impose his or her will upon another. Parents need to make sure their children know that laws stand behind their right to say no and that they have a right to protect themselves against this kind of attack.

Some studies suggest that 45-50 percent and sometimes even 70 percent of the rapes in a particular city may be committed by gangs. In these cases, the act becomes one of violent conquest of the woman, with peer pressure causing the attackers to act in ways they might not have attempted on their own. Adolescents are in the highest risk group to be victimized by a gang.[3]

Nearly half of all rape victims seen in hospital emergency rooms are under 18, and 15 percent are under 12. Rape is not just an issue for adult men and women—it affects our children. Perhaps one important thing that parents can do about rape is to encourage our children to treat women as equals. We need to teach our sons that women are not objects to be victimized when a man wishes to display his power. Even today, rape is used by some soldiers as part of the aggressor's weapons for war. We need to teach our children that there are better ways than violence for nations or individuals to solve disagreements and prove their own self-worth.

Violent Words

In reality, only a small percentage of people exert power over others in the form of actual rape. But many people commit a more subtle form of sexual violence using sexual words as a means of aggression. People use sex-related slang words as a tool for hurting or insulting others, especially as a means for expressing anger. The words give the speaker the illusion of control. With them the speaker not only devalues another person but also symbolically violates that person. Sexual gestures become a way to indicate power without having to prove it and also serve as a way of saying, "you can't hurt me because I don't respect you."

When people use sexual innuendo in their jokes, they may be capitalizing on the shock value of mentioning traditional taboos. The humor often comes because people feel uncomfortable or embarrassed with body parts, functions, or even odors, yet want to pretend that they are not. Off-color jokes tend to capitalize on sexual stereotypes, often perpetuating the idea of women as sex objects.

How should parents handle it when their children come home

with dirty words or undesirable jokes? In our family, we tell the children that there are some words which are not acceptable. Even if we have seen them displayed in public places or heard them on television or in the movies, it is probably not wise to use them. We ask our children if they know the real meaning of the word or understand the joke (often they don't), and then we discuss why people would say that. We suggest that it is usually best to avoid using words in conversation if we don't know their meaning. We talk about how children and adults sometimes use unacceptable words to impress others, but that such speech is often a sign of immaturity instead. We don't condemn anyone for using this language, but try not to use such words ourselves and suggest that there are usually more positive word choices. We stress that our words should be affirming and uplifting, not ways of putting people down. If children feel sad because someone has called them a dirty name, we talk about the fact that words can't change the value of who we are inside.

The Glossary at the conclusion of this book includes some street terms, slang expressions, and euphemisms after the definition of the appropriate word. Although some persons may find the inclusion of these words offensive, we believe that it is essential for parents to be equipped to handle a child's question about words they encounter written on the walls of a public restroom, spoken in a movie, or printed in a book. We have not included these words because we support their use, but specifically because we too find them inappropriate, offensive, and often hate-filled and demeaning.

Sex in the Media

One prominent feature of our society is the role which the media plays in shaping and identifying our values. Almost every American home has at least one television set, and many family members spend 30 hours or more per week watching it. Television has become a cultural institution of our time—what is seen on TV serves as the standard for judging the quality and reality of life. It suggests how we should think, what we should value, and how we should look and behave. If a person's impression of life does not fit the image portrayed by TV, the television is often viewed as the one to trust.

Television programming makes strong statements about sexuality. A majority of primary characters are white, unmarried, middle class males. These men are powerful and often violent. Women are slender, beautiful, and usually dressed in expensive clothes. Intimate sexual interactions are shown or alluded to several times per hour during prime time, with intercourse between unmarried persons shown seven times more frequently than intercourse between married couples. Single women are pictured as less mature or capable than married women, and prostitution and rape are common themes. Cable television has brought R-rated movies and sexually explicit music videos into the home. The soaps seem to glamorize adultery and divorce.

The commercials on television and in magazines also make claims about the shape sexuality should take. Items are advertised as having the ability to make their purchaser more desirable, and brand names are portrayed as status symbols. Sex is used to sell products, and even the packaging of a product can be sexually suggestive. Commercials tend to perpetuate stereotypes about appropriate behavior for men and women, with women pictured in ads for household cleaners, baby products, and beauty items, but men speaking as the voice of authority for most other items. Commercials tend to convey the view that attractive adults are young. Few advertisements—except for medical products or insurance—show people who are over 50.

Although the portrayal of sexuality in the media may be offensive to some people, its picture of violence is even more disturbing. Children watching TV see their favorite characters settling disagreements with fist-fights and handguns; fast-speed car chases and murders are regular features in many scripts. Many shows and movies depict men using force on women, with the women frequently appearing to enjoy this force.

Researchers have found that children watching violence on TV are more likely to participate in violent behavior themselves. They have also found that men who are exposed to sexually violent movies appear to display a higher degree of aggression towards women. Desensitized by watching scenes of explicit violence against women, both men and women appear to become less sympathetic toward injured or sexually assaulted persons in real life.

On the other hand, research has also found that heavy exposure to nonviolent but sexually explicit movies results in a sharp decrease in aggressive behaviors, not the increase that most people fear. Apparently, persons who view high amounts of sex-related films become bored, rather than excited, by what they see.

Most children watch large amounts of TV, often in the absence of an adult. Parents need to be aware of the messages their children are receiving in their viewing and have a strong obligation to guide their children's TV-watching habits. We have the right to say, "I don't want you watching that; I don't want you to think it is OK for people to hurt one another that way." We also have the opportunity to watch TV or movies with our children and to discuss together the values and attitudes that we see. We can use television as the starting point for talking about sex. Or, we can say, "Let's do something instead of watching TV tonight!" We can make sure our children have access to other information and viewpoints besides those typically portrayed on TV.

Homosexuality

Homosexuality is a difficult and sometimes painful reality of American society. Many people fear, misunderstand, and even hate people who have a sexual preference for persons of their own sex, and these people use verses such as Leviticus 20:13 ("You shall not lie with a man as with a woman") to emphasize their disapproval. Although rarely enforced, laws banning "crimes against nature"— which include male homosexual activities—remain in many states. Socially ostracized and the victims of discrimination, many homosexuals feel the need to conceal their sexual orientation.

Researchers are not yet able to pinpoint or agree upon the causes of homosexuality, but the American Psychiatric Association has removed it from the category of mental illness. Most child development specialists assure parents that childhood homosexual curiosity and sex play do not indicate, determine, or alter basic sexual orientation. A single experience with homosexual behavior does not mean that a person is a homosexual.

No matter what our personal opinion concerning the morality of homosexuality may be, there are some things we can do as parents in relationship to this issue. First of all, we can raise our children to be loving and kind to all persons and can help them to treat everyone with dignity and respect. Second, we can teach our children to avoid judging others on the basis of mannerisms, body build, and speech. We can help them to realize that not all homosexuals are alike, just as not all heterosexuals are alike. We can also dispel current myths, such as the idea that most molesters are male homosexuals when, in fact, over 90 percent of the sexual offenses against children are heterosexual men who victimize girls. Third, we can assure our children that we will always be there for them, that we will never reject them, and that they can feel free to talk with us about their concerns and feelings.

Sexually Transmitted Diseases

Although sexuality is a very private matter, our sexual activity cannot be viewed as exclusively our own business. Over one and a half million people each year are infected by Sexually Transmitted Diseases (STDs), which can cause serious bodily injury and even death. Our nation is threatened by the rapidly growing epidemic of AIDS (Acquired Immune Deficiency Syndrome), which can be sexually transmitted and currently has no cure.

One-fifth of all AIDS patients and over one-half of the persons with other STDs are under 25 years old. We cannot afford to raise youth who are ignorant of the causes and seriousness of these diseases. We have a responsibility to warn our children and to teach them how to keep themselves safe.

The term "safe sex" was coined by the New York Task Force on AIDS. It refers to reasonable ways for protecting ourselves against disease and for keeping from knowingly spreading disease to others. Safe sex means taking precautions: avoid intercourse with someone who is infected; avoid promiscuous or group sex; avoid sex with high-risk individuals (such as intravenous drug users); use condoms and spermacides to reduce the risk of infection; take a shower, using warm water and soap, immediately after having sexual intercourse; be honest about your past sexual behavior; secure medical attention immediately if you suspect that you have contracted an infection; and inform your partner if you are carrying a disease. Sex is safest in relationships where neither person has had intercourse with a different partner.

Parents should be aware that in some areas, as many as one third of the sexually active adolescents were found to have a sexually transmitted disease.[4] Most of these diseases (with the exception of AIDS) are readily treated with antibiotics. Yet many youth, particularly those in states which require adult permission before a teenager may receive treatment, do not secure medical attention. Our children need to be assured that we value their health and that we will provide prompt medical care and support, even if we do not condone their sexual activity.

AIDS. Acquired Immune Deficiency Syndrome is an illness which weakens a person's immune system so that the body cannot fight off infections and certain cancers. Two diseases commonly associated with AIDS are a cancer called Kaposi's sarcoma and a type of pneumonia called Pneumoceptis Carnii.

The virus that causes AIDS is the Human Immunodeficiency Virus (HIV). Most people infected with HIV have no symptoms, although they may experience an enlargement of their lymph nodes, fever, diarrhea, and weight loss. Since it can take years for AIDS to develop, it has not yet been determined if everyone with this virus will get AIDS. HIV is found in body fluids such as semen, blood, cervical secretions, and occasionally in the saliva of infected persons. It enters the bloodstream through cuts in the skin or mucous membranes.

AIDS is transmitted by sexual contact with a person who has the AIDS virus or by sharing needles with an infected person during intravenous drug abuse. Pregnant women who have AIDS may give the virus to their babies. HIV has been transmitted through blood transfusions, but blood banks in the United States have eliminated this risk by screening donors and by testing all donated blood for the presence of HIV antibodies. AIDS is not transmitted by casual contact. A person can not pick up the virus from toilet seats, swimming pools, doorknobs, or drinking cups. There is no evidence that mosquitos or pets other than chimpanzees can carry the disease.

From 1981, when AIDS first came to the attention of the American public, until February 1987, a total of 30,396 deaths were attributed to AIDS in the United States. At the time of this writing, there were more than 50,000 reported cases of AIDS, with the World Health Organization estimating as many as 10 million persons worldwide infected with HIV.

In the U.S., male homosexuals have had the highest rate of infection, followed by intravenous drug abusers. It is also possible to contract AIDS through heterosexual contacts. In some countries there are more heterosexuals than homosexuals with AIDS. The disease is rare among children, although 571 cases in children under 13 were reported in the U.S. by September 1987.[5]

Children can be protected from getting diseases such as AIDS by being taught never to pick up hypodermic needles that they see lying around, never to use intravenous drugs, and never to participate in "blood brother or sister ceremonies" by cutting or pricking their fingers and sharing the blood. They should be taught to say "No" if a grown-up wants to touch the private parts of their bodies.

Older children should be taught that the best way to be safe from AIDS is to avoid risky behavior. Affirm their decisions not to become sexually active and not to use illicit drugs. All youth need to know, however, that they should use condoms if they decide to become sexually active and that they should avoid sexual practices that could damage body tissues (such as anal intercourse).

There is currently no cure for AIDS. Experimental drugs are being tested. Scientists are also attempting to develop a vaccine against the AIDS virus, but have not yet been successful.

Recent interviews with women on college campuses have found that many girls do not want to offend their partner by asking him to wear a condom. It appears that they find it easier to risk the possibility of catching a deadly disease than to risk the displeasure of a male. Parents must teach both their sons and daughters that they can stand up for themselves without embarrassment. We must teach our children to be assertive and to have a strong self-esteem that values self-preservation over the approval of someone else. We must also teach our children that selfishness and pride are no reasons to endanger the life of another person.

Gonorrhea. Gonorrhea is an STD disease which has been known for thousands of years. The term was used as early as 140 B.C.

Gonorrhea is caused by a tiny bacteria which cannot survive outside the human body for more than a few seconds. The first symptoms appear three to five days following sexual contact with an infected person. Symptoms include a discharge from the penis or vagina; an extremely painful, burning sensation during urination; and redness, inflammation, and irritation in the genital area.

Untreated gonorrhea can spread through the reproductive system and cause sterility, can enter the bloodstream and spread to the spine, joints, or heart. Blindness can be caused if the bacteria come into contact with the eye. The silver nitrate solution put into the eyes of newborns after birth is to prevent this disease from being passed from an infected mother to her baby during childbirth. Gonorrhea can usually be treated with large doses of penicillin.

Syphilis. In the early stages of the disease, syphilis bacteria cause skin lesions at the point of contact—the external sex organs, the vagina, urethra, anus, mouth, or breasts. During the second stage of the disease, the person may develop a rash, high fever, severe headaches, sore throat, and loss of hair. Eventually, from two to twenty-five years after the infection, the bacteria may attack almost any organ of the body and form lesions in the bones, joints, eyes, mouth, and throat. Persons who are not treated may experience loss of muscle control, paralysis, blindness, deafness, heart disease, or insanity, and may even die.

Congenital syphilis can be transferred from an infected pregnant woman to her baby, causing death or birth defects. Many states have laws which require testing for syphilis before a couple can obtain a marriage license, or during the early months of pregnancy.

Penicillin is virtually 100 percent effective as a treatment for syphilis, especially if taken within one to two hours after contact. Clortetracycline and Oxytetracycline are also effective.

Genital Herpes (Herpes Simplex Type II). Another sexually transmitted disease is Genital Herpes. Caused by a virus which remains for life in the body of the individual, this disease causes tiny blisters in the genital area. Women with herpes are more susceptible to cervical cancer, and the disease can cause severe brain damage and death to babies. No cure has yet been found, although the drug Acyclovir shortens the period of infection.

Chlamydia. Chlamydia trachomatis is a sexually transmitted disease that causes genital infections in men and women. If untreated, chlamydia can cause pelvic infections, miscarriage, and infertility. Chlamydia occurs at a very high rate in the United States. 1984 figures estimate that in some areas of the country, as many as one-third of all sexually active teens were infected with the disease. Chlamydia can be treated with antibiotics.

Trichomoniasis. Trichomoniasis is an infection which causes vaginal discharge and irritation, and may infect the urethra, bladder, and Bartholin glands. As many as one fourth of all gynecological patients in the U.S. have this infection. Males can also be infected, although they usually develop little discomfort from the disease. Trichomoniasis can be transmitted by sexual intercourse, as well as by bath water or unchlorinated swimming pools, or by sharing towels. The infection can be treated with Metronidazole.

Unwanted Pregnancies

Sexual intercourse can have other consequences besides the chance of catching a disease. The most obvious, of course, is pregnancy. Some teenage pregnancies are accidents, some are not. Many adolescents lack a clear understanding of the emotional and economic effects of pregnancy and parenthood. According to statistics by the Alan Guttmacher Institute in 1981, there are nearly 1.25 million teenage pregnancies in the United States each year. Many young women are sexually active, yet nationwide surveys have consistently found that half or more of these girls use contraceptives only occasionally or not at all. Some girls admit their belief that they could not become pregnant the first time they had intercourse.

There are risks to both the mother and the baby when the mother is young. Babies of teenage mothers tend to have a lower birth weight. They are generally weaker, more susceptible to health problems, and may have improperly developed organs and mental disabilities. Teenage mothers tend to have more difficult deliveries and a higher rate of death due to childbirth complications.

There are currently almost three million children under the age of five who were born to teenage mothers. Many of these families are living in poverty or are on welfare. Both unwed mothers and teens who decide to marry have difficulty finishing their schooling and obtaining sufficient funds to provide for their children. Two out of every three pregnant teenagers drop out of school. The divorce rate for couples who marry during their teens is very high.

Parents need to encourage their sons and daughters to *think* before engaging in sexual activity. Have they thought through the possible consequences? What plans have they made for birth control? What do they intend to do if pregnancy occurs? Will they get married? put the child up for adoption? have an abortion? Will the mother try to raise the baby on her own, or expect her parents to help? Are they aware of the costs of rasising a baby or the time and attention that young children require and deserve? Would they be willing to sacrifice their education and their dreams, if necessary, for the sake of a child?

It is obvious that a teenager will not stop to answer all of these questions when he or she is caught up in a moment of sexual excitement. That is why it is important to have talked about these kinds of questions early during the growing-up years. Even older grade school children can think seriously about the consequences of pregnancy, although they may not be able to understand the emotional aspects that would be involved. If they have been encouraged to think about the subject while they are still young, they will hopefully continue to think when they are older.

One way to encourage children to think about sexual matters might be when you are talking about other people. Are there students in your neighborhood who are pregnant? Do you know a boy who is thinking about dropping out of school? Do you know someone who has recently adopted an infant? Is there a relative in your family who "had to get married?" Talking over other people's predicaments can be an opportunity to think through your values and plan how to avoid similar circumstances.

Special Needs and Problems of Exceptional Children

The parents of exceptional children need to remember that their son or daughter is also a sexual being, just like every other boy or girl. Mentally and physically handicapping conditions do not rule out sexual feelings. The need for touch, warmth, tenderness, and intimacy remains, as does the need for sex education. Assure children with handicapping conditions that their bodies are OK. Persons with mental handicaps may function at a childlike level, but have adult sexual desires. Ask about sex education materials that are specially designed for the exceptional child. One such course called "My Body and My Self" is part of the *Living in Faith: A Resource for Teachers of Older Youth and Young Adults Who Are Retarded* (Graded Press).

Like a Deer Prancing Into a Trap

Proverbs 7 tells the colorful story of an inexperienced and foolish young man who was not aware of the difficult sexual situations that exist in the world. Naive and unprepared, he was easily seduced by a beautiful but shameless woman.

> She threw her arms around the young man, kissed
> him, looked him straight in the eye, and
> said . . . "Come on! Let's make love all night

long. . . " Suddenly he was going with her like an ox
on the way to be slaughtered, like a deer prancing
into a trap where an arrow would pierce its heart.
He was like a bird going into a net—he did not
know that his life was in danger.

                                   Proverbs 7:13,18,22-23

The world in which our children live is a world of potential sexual
danger. Our son or daughter may be walking nonchalantly through
life, only to be caught off guard by a problem like sexual abuse, rape,
AIDS, or an unplanned pregnancy. A problem like that could be
devastating—even life destroying! This is not what we want for our
children. We want them to be safe, happy, secure, and to affirm the
blessings of sexuality. But this safety and security does not just
happen. We must be purposeful about preparing our children for
life. As parents, we have a responsibility to see that our children are
informed, aware, and able to protect themselves. Life will always
have dangers, but if our children are prepared, they will be able to
cope and to keep a positive perspective on what it means to be male
or female.

What Caused the Problem?

The list of difficulties associated with human sexuality calls us to
stop and consider: what is the cause of sex-related problems?
Throughout history, people have seldom dealt realistically with the
possibility that relationships are both loving and sexual. From the
very beginning of recorded history, it appears that we have either
idealized or ignored sexuality as a part of life. We have either so
flaunted sexuality that it lost all of its mystery or so covered it up that
all of its beauty was hidden in guilt.

The latter seems to characterize the early Greeks and Romans.
Philosophers in these cultures viewed sexual desire as irrational and
immature. This made it difficult for a person who felt sexual urges to
achieve both pleasure and self-respect. Women in particular were
not supposed to enjoy sex. Couples did not marry for love, but for
the purpose of having children. This attitude was reflected in
doctrines of the early Christian Church in which the leaders wrote
that to enjoy sex was sinful, even within marriage. In the Middle
Ages, "courtly love" became the fashion. Courtly love was tender

and passionate, but not consummated with sexual intercourse. It was thought to make lovers noble, and had no association with marriage. Marriages then, as in many parts of the world today, were arranged by parents on the basis of economic necessity.

During the Victorian era in England (1837-1910), anything with a remote association to sex was considered undiscussable. A person could not talk about eating a "breast" of chicken—you had to call it "white meat." Piano and table legs were covered with fabric to discourage the sexual excitement one might feel in response to looking at the furniture! People began eating "anti-aphrodisiacs" to suppress sexual impulse. For example, Sylvester Graham invented graham crackers, claiming that the wholesomeness of this food would reduce sexual desire.

The early Hebrews did not escape these feelings of guilt and embarrassment, either. For example, women had to "purify" themselves after their menstrual period and after childbirth, so even these natural occurrences could leave a feeling of having done something wrong. Procreation was seen as an obligation, so if a couple did not produce a child they were failing to fulfill their duty. When a person was infertile or too old to bear children, he or she was believed to be under God's curse, and had no right to sexual pleasure. It could be life-threatening for a Hebrew person to engage in improper sexual behavior. Women caught in the act of adultery were stoned to death. Genesis 38:8-10 tells how a man named Onan was put to death for engaging in coitus interruptus (withdrawing the penis before ejaculation).

This is probably one reason why the Old Testament characters were so concerned and upset with the sinfulness of their neighbors. The Hebrews wanted to raise their children to fear Yahweh and obey God's commandments and to be faithful to their heritage and customs as a people. Their desire for their sons and daughters to grow up and marry other Hebrews was central to their survival as a people. However, the Egyptians who held them as slaves, the tribes they encountered while wandering in the wilderness, and the Assyrians and Babylonians who carried them into exile, all held different attitudes about sexuality. This was particularly true of the resident tribes with whom they reluctantly shared Palestine. Deeply ingrained into these religions was a worship of idols which carried sexual implications and ritual prostitution. Apparently these sexual practices proved to be a powerful recruitment tool, used by the people of Canaan in an attempt to draw the Hebrews to the worship of idols. Parents and prophets in Old Testament times continually had to warn the younger generation against being seduced by or adopting the values and practices of these other cultures and religions.

Today, Christian parents realize that our particular values and opinions on sex are not identical to those of the prevailing culture. Our faith informs the way we feel about homosexuality, abortion, premarital sex, and promiscuity. But youth place great emphasis on the viewpoints and ideals of their friends and heroes. For example, our youth may face tremendous peer pressure to engage in premarital sex, even in their early teens. Television commercials appear to indicate that persons need only buy a car or switch brands of toothpaste or deodorant in order to become sexually appealing. And it is obvious that the sexual attitudes and actions of many movie stars, celebrated athletes, or popular musicians do not represent the sexual expression we wish for our children.

Part of Sex Education Is Learning to Love

Our family subscribes to cable television, and we enjoy watching movies together. Of course, it is almost impossible to find movies that don't make some kind of reference to sex. When our children were younger, (and sometimes even still), they used to play the role of "sexuality censors" for these movies. "Yuk! They're kissing! Close your eyes!" they would demand. Laughing, they would scrunch their eyes shut and try to cover our eyes with their hands, knocking our glasses into the bridge of our noses. It became kind of a game.

But sometimes when there would be a bedroom scene, we would catch the kids peeking at the screen out of the corner of their eyes. "What are they doing?" they would ask. We would tend to say something like, "They are showing that they love one another."

It has become common to call sexual intercourse "making love," even though in some cases the act has little to do with love. The desire for sexual intercourse does not bond persons together unless that desire is coupled with genuine caring and affection. While we realize that sexual experiences are not always expressions of love, we still believe that love is the ideal. To us, one of the purposes of sex education is learning how to integrate love and sexuality. As the world-famous psychoanalyst, Dr. Erich Fromm, says in his book *The Art of Loving*, it is the experience of love that lifts a person from feelings of isolation and aloneness.

> Sexual attraction creates, for the moment, the illusion
> of union, yet without love this union leaves strangers
> as far apart as they were before.[6]

The seventeenth century Puritans were among the first to view sex as a positive bond of pleasure, a gift from God intended to strengthen and enhance marriage. As contemporary Christians, we believe this viewpoint is still valuable and valid and one which we uphold for our children. We want our children to see how actions of love can be beautiful and appropriate ways to express concern and care for another person. As Fromm says, "What does one person give to another?"

> He gives of himself, of the most precious he has, he
> gives of his life. This does not necessarily mean that he
> sacrifices his life for the other, but that he
> gives . . . that which is alive in him: he gives . . . of
> his joy, of his interest, of his understanding, of his
> knowledge, of his humor, of his sadness—of all
> expressions and manifestations of that which is alive
> in him.[7]

Sexuality as an Expression of God's Desire for Humanity

One of the fundamentals of our Christian faith is that we ought to love one another. The ability and desire to care for others is both a gift and a command:

> Dear friends, let us love one another, for love
> comes from God. Whoever loves is a child of God
> and knows God. God is love, and whoever lives in
> love lives in union with God and God lives in
> union with him. There is no fear in love; perfect
> love drives out all fear.
> I John 4:7, 16b-17a, 18a

We were created in the image of God. Genesis 1:27 says that in giving birth to us, God formed a being that is incomplete on its own—a being that needs the touch and warmth of companionship in order to reach its full human potential. To be human is to need relationship and love. Babies need to be held and cuddled in order to thrive. Older adults who are isolated from human contact become depressed, lose touch with reality, and no longer exhibit the will to live. At every age, our yearning to be close to other persons is an expression of our basic need for relationship.

One of the key components of this yearning is our sexuality. Though by gender we are either male or female, we each have a unique interpretation of what it means to be male and what it means to be female. We have individual ways of expressing maleness and femaleness. Yet, despite these interpretations and expressions, the role of sexuality remains the same. Our sexuality is both a symbol and a power. As a symbol it reminds us of our need for others in becoming what God has imagined for us. Created in the image of God, we too are creators—creators of beauty, of relationships, and of new life. As a power, our sexuality draws us ever more deeply into the intimacy where we discover our creative potential and that of our sisters and brothers.

Affirming and expressing our God-given sexuality is a way to understand the indwelling presence of God in our lives. Ours is a passionate God who weeps when estranged, who continues to seek after us, who came to us in the birth of Christ, and who comes to us in the act of Communion as a God of the flesh as well as of the spirit. God enters into our lives in a real and human way, calling us to accept the touch and power of God's love and longing to fill our emptiness and make us whole.

God's desire for humanity is that we should not be separated from God nor from others, for alienation from God and others is life-denying and destructive. Unfortunately, we know that sex can be a vehicle for alienation when it is used to dominate or to limit another, to express hostility, or to cause pain and fear. But this alienation is a result of sexuality misused, of sex used to manipulate and bruise. This kind of sex is aggressive; it kills and destroys not only self-esteem, but also the spirit that binds us into relationships.

God came to us in bodily form that we "might have life—life in all its fullness" (John 10:10). Such a life is accepting of self and affirming of others and recognizes the God-given element of sexuality. It will not be expressed in oppression or dominance, but in vulnerability, openness, and respect. As such, it can be a vehicle for wholeness and joy. It is our great privilege as parents to assist our children in the discovery of such a life.

A Prayer for Parents and Children Living in an Imperfect World:

Loving God, we live in a confusing and dangerous world—
—a world where children are sexually abused, sometimes by the very ones who ought to love them the most;
—a world where the words and acts of intimacy can be distorted into weapons of violence and power;
—a world where children have children, where TV speaks louder than the heart, and where people risk death or disease for a moment of pleasure.
Forgive us, Lord.
Help us to make our world a place of safety, and teach us to embrace sexuality as a source and force of love!
Amen.

CHAPTER 6

SUGGESTED ACTIVITIES FOR GROUP STUDY

Session 1: Hopes and Expectations

1. Ask participants to get into pairs. Have spouses pair with other partners for this exercise. Instruct partners to tell each other some of the hopes, expectations, and worries they have concerning their children. Then, bring the total group back together again. Ask them to introduce their partners and to report one hope and one worry that their partners expressed. Record these responses on a large sheet of paper or on the chalkboard.

After everyone has been introduced, invite the group to study the two lists and to discuss how their hopes and worries relate to the values of our society. Ask them to assist you in identifying which of the items listed are related to issues of sexuality.

2. Ask the participants to prepare a list of topics which they would want to see covered in a sex education course. Ask the group which of these elements they have already discussed with their children. How was this done? Which were the most easy and which were most difficult?

3. Divide participants into two groups, and ask each group to create a scenario for a typical family evening. One group should picture a positive family atmosphere, where the self-esteem of family members is affirmed; the other should picture a negative family atmosphere. Have each group act out its scenario. Then read Philippians 2:1-4. Discuss the factors that contribute to a positive atmosphere and how a family can intentionally build self-esteem.

4. Ask the group, "What things have you done as a family, or what things do you plan to do, to help your children know God? How did your parents help you in this area? What things did *they* do better, and what things are *you* doing better? Why?"

5. Divide participants into the same two groups that you used for exercise 3—a "negative" family and a "positive" family—and tell them that they are to roleplay conversations that might take place in their family. The "positive" family should demonstrate ways in which parents can encourage communication and good listening; the "negative family" should employ communication "stoppers."

Possible situations:
- child says, "I hate school!"
- parent asks child to clean room, but child doesn't do it
- child bites his sister on the arm
- child wants to buy an expensive toy or outfit

6. Pray together the Prayer of Hope and Expectation, page 15.

Session 2: Knowing, Deciding, and Being in Control

1. Ask the participants to think back to their childhood and to consider what were the most important decisions that they had to make when they were four years old, eight years old, and twelve years old. Ask participants how they made those decisions and if they would be satisfied if their children would use the same decision-making process. Why or why not?

2. Work with the group to develop a list of some decisions and choices that are appropriate for a child to make at each of these three age levels. Record their responses on a large sheet of paper. Group members might not be in agreement, so discuss with them why they do or do not (or why they would or would not) allow their children to make these decisions.

3. Play one of the object games described on pages 19-20 of chapter 1. Discuss with the group how such games can help children learn to think and to be aware of their surroundings.

4. Divide the participants into small groups of two or three persons. Instruct each group to pick a personal value that they hold—one they would like to pass on to their children. Ask, "What might a parent do to communicate this value to his or her child? Try to think of at least five different ways." Bring the group back together again and have the small groups report their conclusions.

5. Read Exodus 2:11–3:6 for the group. Ask, "What were the self-control issues in this passage? Can we say Moses shows self-control? What might have happened had he acted differently?"

6. Roleplay a number of situations where being able to say no is important. Some examples:
- a boy pressuring a girl for sex
- a boss pressuring an employee to do something unethical
- a child being dared to break into a vacant house

Ask the class participants to observe which strategies were successful and which were not.

7. Pray together the Prayer for Clarity of Thought, page 27.

Session 3: Understanding Our Child's Sexuality

1. Ask group members to recall and discuss their earliest memories of being a boy or a girl or how old they were when they first became aware of their gender.

2. Give participants each a small piece of paper and a pencil. Ask them to write down an action or behavior that they feel would be a sexually inappropriate behavior for a child. Collect the slips, read each one, and have the group talk about whether they agree that this would be inappropriate. Invite participants to discuss how they determine what is appropriate. Encourage participants to suggest ways a parent might handle that particular situation.

3. Assign an age level—before birth, birth-1 year, 1-2 years, 3-5 years, 6-8 years, 9-12 years—to each participant. Ask the persons assigned to each level to make a chart on one or more large sheets of paper describing their perceptions of the differences between boys and girls at that age level and listing how children of that age experience sexuality. Have them choose a symbol for children at their particular age level.

Come together as a large group to discuss the charts and symbols. Summarizing the material found in chapter 3, add to the charts as they are presented to the group. You may also wish to contribute details based on memories of yourself as a child or personal observations about your own children or children you know.

4. Ask participants to each think of a child that they know quite well. Based on their perceptions of these children and their developmental levels, the participants are to list three specific things that they might do to enhance that child's sexual identity. Ask participants to find partners who have chosen a child from the same age level and to compare their plans.

5. Ask participants to each read quickly through Genesis 25:25-34 and 27:1-45 and to discuss what parenting advice they would have given to Isaac and Rebekah.

6. Close by reading Psalm 127:3-5 and by praying together the Prayer for Understanding, page 51.

Session 4: The Question Box

1. Open by reading Ephesians 4:29. Divide the group into twos or threes. Ask ask them to respond to and discuss these questions:

- What was the most unpleasant experience you had as a child when talking about sex with your parents?
- What was best experience you had as a child when talking about sex with your parents?
- What has been the most embarrassing time and place that your children have asked you something about sex?

2. Have the women and the men form separate groups. Ask them to discuss whether or not they agree with the statement that fathers are less likely than mothers to talk about sex with their children. Ask them to consider why this might be true and to suggest ways that fathers might be encouraged to become more involved with sex education. Bring the total group back together and discuss your suggestions. Point out ways in which the women's ideas on this subject differ from the men's.

3. Invite the group to think of "avoidance" words or phrases—words people use instead of the proper terms when they are talking about embarrassing sexual subjects. Some examples are "in a family way," "sleeping together," and "going to the bathroom." Next, ask them to think of slang expressions related to sex—all of the "dirty words") that they can think of. Lead the group in a discussion of their feelings with regards to the use of these words and, in contrast, their feelings about using the proper terminology.

4. Ask the participants to think about the past week and to identify some experiences that they either used or might have used as teachable moments. Invite participants to talk about some of these incidents, to evaluate whether or not they used these occasions to their best advantage as teachable moments, and to consider what they might do differently if the same situation came up again.

5. Practice answering children's questions about sex. Ask volunteers to give their own answers to some of the questions listed on pages 59-73 of chapter 4. Invite participants to suggest questions that are not in the book. Allow volunteers to offer their answers.

6. Read Proverbs 4 and pray the Prayer for Wisdom, page 75.

Session 5: The Real World

1. Read to the group the statistics found in the section titled "Sexual Abuse of Children" on pages 77-78 of chapter 5. Ask participants to raise their hands if they know someone who has been sexually abused. Discuss whether or not the national statistics appear to be consistent with the experience of the participants.

2. Divide participants into small groups of three to six persons in each group. Ask each group to plan a puppet skit that might be used with children, teaching them how to be protected against sexual abuse. Make puppets, using craft materials such as paper plates, old socks, small paper bags, crayons or felt-tip markers, buttons, yarn, and so forth. Have each group present their skit. When all skits have been presented, ask participants to point out ways each skit might be effective in communicating with children. Invite the group to discuss the possibility of presenting these skits to their children or to the children of the whole church.

3. Divide participants into three groups. Assign each group one of the following passages: 2 Samuel 13; Genesis 34; Judges 19–21. Ask each group to discuss the relationship of rape and violence as portrayed in their assigned passages and to compare how the crime of rape was viewed in biblical times with how it is viewed today.

4. If you have access to a television, turn it on, and watch for five to seven minutes, changing the channel every minute and a half or so. Give each participant a sheet of paper and a pencil and ask them to write down everything they see that has a sexual implication. Turn off the television and discuss the influence that the media has on our values, especially in relationship to sex. An option to this activity would be to prepare a videotape of short clips from commercials and then to proceed with the same format for discussion.

5. Discuss the sections on Sexually Transmitted Diseases (STD's), Acquired Immune Deficiency Syndrome (AIDS), and Unwanted Pregnancies found on pages 86-91. Ask for volunteers to explain the specific methods they have used or have thought about using with their children to discuss these difficult topics. Consider the following: What did the children want to know? What did you (the parent) say? What caused particular discomfort? What do you think have been the results of your conversation?

6. Read Genesis 1:27 and 31 and 1 John 4:7, 16b–17a, and 18a to the group. Ask, "What do you think these passages have to say about the relationship between God and human sexuality? What are some ways that our sexuality can help us to understand God? What other Bible passages have influenced your personal feelings and attitudes about sexuality?"

7. Ask the participants to read Proverbs 7:6–27 silently. Then ask them to spend several moments in silent prayer, asking for God's guidance and protection for their child. Pray together the Prayer for Parents and Children Living in an Imperfect World, page 97.

ENDNOTES

Chapter 3:

1. John Money, *Love and Love Sickness: The Science of Sex, Gender Difference and Pair Bonding*. Baltimore: Johns Hopkins University Press, 1980.
2. Judith Rich Harris and Robert M. Liebert, *The Child*, Englewood Cliffs, New Jersey: Prentice-Hall, Inc., 1984.
3. M. Ainsworth, M.L. Blehar, E. Waters and S. Wall. *Patterns of Attachment*, Hissdale, New Jersey: Erlbaum, 1978.
4. M. Louise Biggar, "Maternal Aversion to Mother-Infant Contact," *The Many Facets of Touch, The Foundation of Experience: Its Importance Through Life, With Initial Emphasis for Infants and Young Children*, Johnson and Johnson, 1984, pp. 66-74.
5. Anneliese Korner, "The Many Faces of Touch," *The Many Facets of Touch*, Johnson and Johnson, 1984, pp. 107-113.
6. E.H. Erikson, *Childhood and Society*, 2nd Edition, New York: Norton, 1963.
7. E.E. Maccoby and C.N. Jacklin. *The Psychology of Sex Difference*, Standford, California: Standford University Press, 1974.
8. L. Shapio, "A Study of Peer Groups Interaction in 8 and 28 Month Old Children," Ph.D. Dissertation, Harvard University, 1969.
9. J.W.M. Whiting and B. Whiting, cited in W. Mischel's "Sex Sterotyping and Socialization," *Carmichael's Manual of Child Psychology*, Vol. 2, 3rd Ed., New York: Wiley, 1970.
10. Sandra Weiss, "The Language of Touch: A Resource to Body Image," *Issues in Mental Health Nursing*, Vol. 1, pp. 17-29, 1978.

Chapter 4:

1. Susan M. Bennett, "Family Environment for Sexual Learning as a Function of Father's Involvement in Family Work and Discipline," *Adolescence*, Vol. XIX, No. 75, Fall, 1984, pp. 609-627.

Chapter 5:

1. Paul C. Vance, "Love and Sex—Can We Talk About That at School?", *Childhood Education*, Vol. 61, No. 4, March/April 1985, pp. 272-276.
2. Patricia Beezley Mrazek and C. Henry Kempe. *Sexually Abused Children and Their Families*, New York: Pergamon Press, 1981, pp. 91-92, 230.
3. Robert Coles and Geoffrey Stokes, *Sex and the American Teenager*, New York: Harper Colophon Books, 1985, pp. 108-110.
4. David A. Schulz, *Human Sexuality*, Englewood Cliffs, New Jersey: Prentice Hall, 1988, p. 347.
5. U.S. Department of Health and Human Services, Public Health Service. Centers for Disease Control.
6. Erich Fromm, *The Art of Loving*, New York: Harper and Row, 1956, p. 46.
7. Erich Fromm, op. cit., p. 20.

RECOMMENDED RESOURCES

Books for Adults:

Embodiment: An Approach to Sexuality and Christian Theology, by James B. Nelson, (Augsburg, 1979). A theological look at human sexuality; (ISBN 0-8066-1701-2) $12.95

The Family Book About Sexuality, by Mary Calderone and Eric Johnson (Harper and Row, 1981). Designed to be used by family members of all ages; (ISBN 0-690-01910-6) $14.95.

How to Talk With Your Child About Sexuality, by Faye Wattleton and Susan Newcomer (Planned Parenthood Federation of America, 1986). A practical and straightforward guide for parents of preschoolers through teens; (ISBN 0-385-18443-3) $7.95.

Straight Talk: Sexuality Education for Parents and Kids 4-7, by Marilyn Ratnner and Susan Chamlin (Penquin, 1987). Contains "Kid's Place"—a pull-out section of activities for children; (ISBN 0-14-009413-X) $4.95.

What to Tell Your Child About Sex, revised edition, by the Child Study Association of America (Aronson, 1983). Discusses sexual development in children up to age 17; (ISBN 0-87668-708-7) $15.00.

Books for Children:

A Better Safe Than Sorry Book, by Sol and Judith Gordon (Ed-U Press, 1986). Designed to teach children aged three through nine how to prevent sexual assault; (ISBN 0-934978-13-1) $7.95.

Are You There, God? It's Me, Margaret, by Judy Blume (Dell, 1986). A novel about a girl's anxieties over puberty; (ISBN 0-440-40419-3) $2.95.

Created by God: About Human Sexuality for Older Girls and Boys, by Dorlis Brown Glass with James H. Ritchie, Jr. (Graded Press, 1989). A reading book for older elementary children that doubles as a curriculum resource for group study; emphasizes Christian values, responsibility, relationships, and self-esteem along with comprehensive anatomical and physiological information; (ISBN 0-687-75345-7) $1.85.

Did the Sun Shine Before You Were Born?, by Sol and Judith Gordon

(Ed-U Press, 1982). Exceptional realistic illustrations that include multi-racial and handicapped children; (ISBN 0-934978-03-4) $7.95.

Facts About Sex for Today's Youth, by Sol Gordon (Ed-U Press, 1985). Brief; easy reading (fourth and fifth grade level); (ISBN 0-934978-01-8) $7.95.

How Babies are Made, by Andrew C. Andry and Steven Schepp (Little, 1984). The story of reproduction in plants, animals, and humans; (ISBN 0-316-04227-7) $7.70.

I'll Get There: It Better Be Worth the Trip, by John Donovan (Harp J., 1969). A novel dealing with homosexuality; (ISBN 0-06-021718-9) $12.89.

It's Not What You'd Expect, by Norma Klein (Avon, 1982). A novel which deals with an extramarital affair; (ISBN 0-380-00011-3) $2.50.

A Little Demonstration Of Affection, by Elizabeth Winthrop (Harp J., 1975). A novel which raises the issue of incest; (ISBN 0-06-026558-2) $11.89.

Love and Sex in Plain Language, by Eric W. Johnson (Lippincott, 1977). Informative book for 10-12 year olds which stresses personal responsibility; (ISBN 0-397-01231-4) $12.25.

Making Babies. An Open Family Book., by Sara Bonnett Stein (Walker, 1974). Discusses the importance of an open family atmosphere; has two texts—one for young children, another for adults; (ISBN 0-8027-7221-8) $7.95.

The Man Without A Face, by Isabelle Holland (Harp J., 1987). A novel which deals with homosexuality; (ISBN 0-694-05611-1) $2.95.

Mom, the Wolfman & Me, by Norma Klein (Avon, 1982). A novel which deals with an extramarital affair; (ISBN 0-380-01725-3) $2.50.

No More Secrets for Me, by Oralee Wachter (Little, Brown, 1984). Four separate stories of children who are touched in ways they do not want to be touched; a sensitive treatment of a difficult subject; (ISBN 0-316-91491-6) $4.70.

Then Again, Maybe I Won't, by Judy Blume (Dell, 1986). A novel about the problems faced by adolescent boys; (ISBN 0-440-48659-9) $2.95.

The What's Happening to My Body? Book for Boys: A Growing Up Guide for Parents and Sons, by Lynda Madaras with Dane Saavedra; and *The What's Happening to My Body? Book for Girls: A Growing Up Guide for Parents and Daughters*, by Lynda Madaras with Area Madaras (Newmarket Press, 1987). Two very comprehensive books that answer the questions children and youth have about their bodies; (ISBN 0-937858-99-4 /girls 0-937858-98-6 /boys) $9.95.

Where Do Babies Come From?, by Margaret Sheffield (Knopf, 1973). Excellent illustrations; direct and accurate terminology; (ISBN 0-394-48482-7) $10.95.

Films, Filmstrips, and Videos:

Better Safe Than Sorry (Vitascope-Filmfair, 1987). VHS/Beta, color, 17 minutes. 2nd edition. Stresses a child's responsibility for his or her own safety. $40 to rent; $345 to purchase.

Better Safe Than Sorry II (Vitascope-Filmfair, 1983). VHS/Beta, color, 15 minutes. Presents simple rules to help children prevent sexual abuse. $30 to rent, $260 to purchase.

Both videos available from Filmfair, 10900 Ventura, P.O. Box 1728, Studio City, CA 91604.

A Family Talks About Sex (Perennial, 1978). 16mm film, color, 29 minutes. Designed to help parents communicate. Available from EcuFilm; $20 to rent.

Children and Sexuality (Graded Press, 1989) VHS, color, 30 minutes. Developed as a companion video to this book. David Elkind helps parents and teachers prepare to teach children a Christian view of sexuality. $24.95.

Kids Who Have Kids are Kidding Themselves (Educational Activities, 1979) 35mm filmstrip, color. Encourages responsibility in relationships. Available from Educational Activities, Box 392, Freeport, NY 11520; $39 to purchase.

New Image Teen Theatre (Planned Parenthood of San Diego, 1985). VHS, color, 30 minutes. Dramatizes communication on sexuality; winner of Alpha Award for Excellence in Children's Programming. Available from Printed Matter, Inc.; P.O. Box 15246; Atlanta, GA 30333. $20 to rent; $90 to purchase.

Sex: A Topic for Conversation With Dr. Sol Gordon (Mondell Productions, 1987). VHS/Beta. Three videos—for parents of young children, parents of teenagers, and for teenagers themselves. Humorous, using a question-and-answer format. Available from Mondell Productions; 5215 Homer St.; Dallas, TX 75206. rental, $49 each; for purchase $99 each or $250 for all three.

GLOSSARY

Included parenthetically in the following definitions are some of the street terms, slang expressions, and euphemisms commonly used in reference to human anatomy and sexual behaviors. We find the use of many such expressions offensive and demeaning, especially when terms related to sexual intercourse double as ways of speaking about acts of violence or are used to verbally abuse others. The words included are ones your children will encounter on the street, at school, on television, in movies, or on the walls of public restrooms. Adults who understand the meaning of these words can direct their children to proper terminology and can help their children adopt a more Godly, loving attitude toward sex and sexuality. There is also a self-esteem issue raised: children will feel better about themselves if they know what words mean—even words that they have no intention of using.

abortion. The surgical removal of an embryo or fetus from a pregnant woman's uterus before the embryo or fetus is able to survive on its own.

Acquired Immune Deficiency Syndrome (AIDS). A disease caused by the Human Immunodeficiency Virus (HIV). AIDS causes the breakdown of the body's immune system, making it impossible for the body to fight off other diseases. AIDS is transmitted by the exchange of body fluids—primarily through sexual intercourse but also through the sharing of needles by drug users and from infected mothers to their babies.

adolescence. The period of life extending from the beginning of puberty to adulthood.

amniocentesis (AM-nee-oh-sen-TEE-sis). The surgical insertion of a hollow needle through a woman's abdominal wall and into the uterus to obtain a sample of the amniotic fluid. This process is used to check for birth defects in a developing fetus.

amnion (AM-nee-ahn). The thin membrane sac filled with a watery solution called amniotic fluid that surrounds and protects the developing fetus in its mother's uterus.

ampulla (am-POOL-uh). The flared-out portion of the vas deferens near the prostate gland, where sperm are stored until ejaculated.

androgen. A hormone that influences growth and the sex drive in males. It is responsible for sex characteristics such as voice change and hair growth.

anus. The opening in the rectum for the expulsion of solid waste—feces—from the body. (ass hole)

artificial insemination. The introduction of semen into the vagina of a woman by means other than sexual intercourse in an attempt to overcome fertility problems.

athletic supporter. An elastic strap worn around the pelvic area by men and boys during strenuous exercise. Supports and protects the testicles by holding them close to the body. Commonly known as a jock strap.

bartholin glands. Two small, oval-shaped glands in the female that produce a lubricating fluid in the vaginal area.

Basal Body Temperature (BBT). A technique for determining female ovulation by observing changes in body temperature upon awakening each morning.

birth control. Preventing conception from taking place.

birth control pill. A medication that prevents ovulation and therefore prevents pregnancy. Medication must be taken exactly as prescribed in order to be effective. Often referred to as the pill.

bisexuality. Being sexually active with or sexually attracted to persons of both sexes. (AC/DC)

breasts. Two glands on the upper chest of both males and females, the growth of which is stimulated at puberty. In females, the breasts develop so that they are able to produce milk at the birth of a baby. (boobs, jugs, knockers, melons, tits)

caesarian section. Delivery of a baby by surgical incision through the abdomen into the uterus.

cervix (SIR-viks). The lower, narrow portion of the uterus which connects with the vagina.

chancre (SHANG-kuhr). A sore or ulcerated area, usually on the genitals, that appears during the early stage of syphilis.

chlamydia (KLUH-mid-ee-uh). A bacteria-caused STD that is a particular problem for females due to the lack of external symptoms. A woman can appear healthy while the disease is spreading infection and seriously damaging the uterus, fallopian tubes, and ovaries.

chromosome. The DNA-containing structure in the nucleus of a cell which serves as the carrier of genes and genetic information.

circumcision. The surgical removal of the foreskin—the loose layer of skin that extends over the glans or head of the penis—for hygenic, religious, or cosmetic reasons.

clitoris (KLIT-uh-ris). The small, cylinder-shaped, highly sensitive female organ located at the top of the inner labia. It corresponds to the penis in males. (clit, pea)

conceive. To become pregnant.

conception. The fertilization of the female ovum by the male sperm, which marks the beginning of pregnancy.

condom. A thin sheath, usually of rubber or latex, placed on the erect penis before sexual intercourse to prevent the spread of disease and/or to prevent sperm from entering the vagina. Also called a prophylactic. (rubber, safe)

cunnilingus (kuhn-uh-LING-guhs). Using the mouth to stimulate the vulva and vagina. (eating)

diaphragm. A soft rubber dome that is filled with a spermicide and inserted into the vagina before sexual intercourse.

douche. The cleansing of the vagina with a liquid solution or water.

ejaculation. The discharge of semen from the penis in a series of intense muscle contractions during orgasm. (come)

embryo. An unborn human from about the tenth day after conception until the third month of pregnancy.

endometrium (ehn-doh-MEE-tree-uhm). The uterine lining that thickens and fills with blood in preparation to receive a fertilized ovum.

epididymis (ep-uh-DID-uh-mihs). The mass of tiny tubes where sperm cells mature. It is attached to the back portion of the testicle.

erection. The enlargement and hardening of the penis or clitoris as tissues fill with blood, usually in response to sexual stimulation. (males—boner, hard-on)

erogenous (ih-RAHG-uh-nuhs) **zones.** Areas of the body that are especially sensitive to sexual stimulation, including the mouth, lips, breasts, nipples, anus, and genitals.

estrogen. The female sex hormone that is produced primarily in the ovaries and is responsible for the development of secondary sex characteristics such as breast development and widened hips.

fallopian (fa-LOH-pee-uhn) **tubes.** The two tubes through which the ova pass from the ovaries to the uterus.

fellatio (fuh-LAY-she-oh). Oral stimulation of the penis. (blow job, sucking off)

fertility. The condition of being able to produce offspring.

fertilization. The union of the sperm cell nucleus with the nucleus of the ovum to start a new baby. Also called conception.

fetus. An unborn human from about the third month of pregnancy until birth.

foreplay. Any type of sex play that precedes and prepares persons for sexual intercourse.

foreskin. The extension of loose skin that covers the glans or head of a male's penis at birth. Its removal for hygenic, religious, or cosmetic reasons is called circumcision.

gay. A homosexual person; more specifically, a male homosexual.

gender. Being male or female.

genital herpes (HER-peez). An incurable, virus-caused STD. In females it can lead to cancer of the cervix. The chief symptom is painful, blister-like sores that surface periodically for the remainder of the infected person's life.

genitals. The external male and female sex organs—the penis, scrotum, and testicles in males, and the vulva in females. (privates)

gestation. The period between conception and birth. Also called pregnancy.

gonads (GOH-nadz). The reproductive cell-producing glands; the testicles in the male and the ovaries in the female.

gonorrhea (gahn-uh-REE-uh). An STD caused by bacteria; can cause blindness, damage to heart and brain, severe arthritis, sterility, and death.

heterosexuality. Being sexually active with or sexually attracted to a person or persons of the other sex. (straight)

homosexuality. Being sexually active with or sexually attracted to a person or persons of one's own sex. (female homosexual: dyke, les; male homosexual: fag, faggot, homo, pansy, queer)

hormones. Chemical substances, produced by glands, that regulate the functioning of other organs.

hymen (HI-muhn). A thin membrane that partially covers the opening to the vagina. It may be torn during strenuous exercise, masturbation, or first sexual intercourse. Some women are born without a hymen. (cherry, maidenhead)

hysterectomy (hiss-tuh-RECK-tuh-mee). Surgical removal of the uterus.

impotence (IHM-puh-tuhns). A male's inability to achieve or maintain an erection during sexual intercourse.

incest. Sexual intercourse between close relatives; a practice forbidden in most cultures.

intercourse. See sexual intercourse.

Intrauterine Device (IUD). A soft plastic or metal birth control device that must be inserted into and removed from the uterus by a doctor. While questions have been raised as to the safety of this means of birth control, it continues in use.

labia (LAY-bee-uh). Two sets of folds of skin that are part of the vulva. The outer or major labia surround the opening to the vagina. The inner or minor labia are inside and sometimes hidden by the outer labia. The word *labia* means "lips."

labor. The stage of giving birth during which the cervix dilates or enlarges, allowing the contractions of the uterine muscles to push the baby from the uterus into the vagina in preparation for delivery.

lesbian. A female homosexual.

masturbation (mass-tuhr-BAY-shuhn). Self-stimulation of one's genitals to create sexual pleasure. (beating off, beating the meat, getting your rocks off, jacking off, jerking off, playing with yourself, whacking off)

menarche (muh-NAHR-kee). The onset of menstruation in females.

menopause (MEHN-uh-pahz). That time in a woman's life—usually between the ages of 45 and 55—during which menstruation ceases and pregnancy is no longer possible. Also referred to as change of life.

menstruation (mehn-STRAY-shun). The discharge of blood, secretions, and tissue from the uterus that females experience about once a month. Also referred to as the period.

miscarriage. The natural expulsion of an embryo or fetus from the uterus before it is mature enough to survive, usually due to some abnormal development. More properly referred to as a spontaneous abortion.

mons pubis (mahns PEW-bihs). The area at the base of the man's abdomen and just above the penis where the pubic bone is located. With the onset of puberty it is covered with hair.

mons veneris (mahns VEHN-uh-riss). The mound of fatty tissue covering the pubic bone at the base of the woman's abdomen, between the thighs. With the onset of puberty it is covered with hair. (bush)

Natural Family Planning (NFP). Women wanting to avoid pregnancy keep charts of daily body temperature and cervical secretions in order to determine when ovulation is to take place. Intercourse is then avoided on certain days.

nocturnal emission. Spontaneous ejaculation of built-up semen that occurs during sleep and is often associated with sexual dreams. Also called a seminal emission or wet dream.

oral sex. Using the mouth to stimulate the genitals.

orgasm. The peak of excitement in sexual activity, resulting in a highly pleasurable series of muscle spasms, and followed by a sudden discharge of accumulated sexual tension.

ovaries. Two almond-sized female reproductive glands in which ova develop and sex hormones are produced.

ovulation (ah-vue-LAY-shuhn). The ripening and release of an ovum from an ovary, usually occurring about once a month.

ovum. The female reproductive cell. The plural is ova.

penis. The cylindrical portion of the male genitals through which urine and semen pass. The primary parts are the shaft, glans or head, and foreskin. It corresponds to the clitoris in females. (cock, dick, meat, pecker, peter, prick, tool, wiener)

period. The time of menstrual flow. (curse, on the rag, that time of the month)

petting. Noncoital sexual activity such as stimulation of the breasts and genitals.

pituitary (pih-TOO-uh-tare-ee) **gland**. An endocrine gland attached to the base of the brain which secretes a number of hormones to control body processes.

placenta (pluh-SEN-tuh). A spongy organ containing a network of blood vessels that develops on the lining of the uterus during pregnancy; it enables the exchange of food, oxygen, and waste materials between mother and child.

pregnancy. The period from conception to birth. The condition of having a developing embryo or fetus within the female body. (expecting, in a family way, knocked up)

prostate (PROSS-tate) **gland**. An organ surrounding the male urethra that secretes part of the seminal fluid. The contraction of the prostate helps to force the semen out through the urethra during ejaculation.

puberty (PEW-bur-tee). The period of rapid development during which the sex organs mature and begin to produce either ova or sperm.

pubic hair. Coarse, curly hair that grows in the genital area.

rape. Forcing someone to have sexual intercourse. (gang bang—rape by multiple assailants)

rectum. The lower end of the large intestine, ending at the anus.

sanitary napkin. A pad of absorbent cotten worn inside the underpants to absorb the menstrual discharge. (rag)

scrotum. The loose pouch of skin in the male, beneath the penis, that contains the testicles, (bag, sack)

semen. The whitish fluid containing sperm, which is ejaculated from the penis during orgasm. Also called seminal fluid. (come, jism)

seminal vesicles. Two small pouches in a male, located at the back of the prostate gland, where semen is produced.

sensuality. The unique combination of elements such as strength, vulnerability, sensitivity, honesty, self-esteem, energy level, and physical appearance that one person perceives and is attracted to in another person.

sex-role stereotypes. Culturally imposed, broad generalizations about particular traits associated with masculinity or femininity.

sexual intercourse. Sexual activity where the penis is inserted into the vagina. Also called coitus or copulation. (balling, banging, doing it, fucking, getting laid, going all the way, making love, scoring, screwing, sleeping together)

sexuality. The sum of a person's sexual orientation, characteristics, and behaviors.

Sexually Transmitted Diseases (STD's). A variety of diseases contracted through sexual activity. These were formerly called veneral disease or VD.

sodomy (SAW-duh-mee). Anal intercourse. The term is also used at times in reference to oral sex or having sexual intercourse with an animal.

sperm. The male reproductive cell.

spermicide. A sperm-killing chemical placed in the vagina prior to sexual intercourse. It comes in the form of creams, jellies, dissolving tablets, aerosol foams, and sponges.

sterility. The inability to produce offspring. Also called infertility. (barren)

sterilization. The surgical process of making an individual permanently incapable of reproduction.

surrogate mother. A woman who is artificially inseminated by sperm from the male of a couple unable to conceive due to the female's infertility or inability to carry a child full term. The surrogate mother carries the child until birth and then gives the child to the couple.

syphilis (SIHF-uh-luhs). An STD caused by a microorganism called a spirochete; the first symptom appears 10-90 days or more after exposure in the form of a sore at the point where the infection entered the body. While the sore will eventually go away, the untreated disease can affect the brain, heart, liver, or bones, and can cause irrreparable birth defects if passed from a mother to her unborn child.

tampon (TAM-pahn). A roll of absorbent material that is inserted into the vagina to absorb the menstrual discharge.

testicles (testes). The egg-shaped male reproductive glands in which sperm and testosterone are produced. They are suspended in a loose pouch of skin between the legs. (balls, family jewels, marbles, nuts, rocks, stones)

testosterone (tess-TOSS-tuh-roan). The male sex hormone, produced primarily in the testicles, which is responsible for the full development of the genitals and the secondary sex characteristics.

transsexual. A person who has a persistent sense of discomfort with his or her biological gender and may choose to undergo surgery to achieve the outward appearance of the other sex.

transvestite. One who derives sexual gratification from dressing in the clothing of the other sex.

tubal ligation (TOO-buhl lie-GAY-shun). A surgical procedure for sterilization in females. The fallopian tubes are cut, tied, sealed, or otherwise blocked off, either through an incision in the abdomen or through the vagina. Ova continue to be produced but they are reabsorbed by the body. Commonly referred to as having one's tubes tied.

umbilical cord. The cord connecting the unborn infant to the placenta through which the fetus receives nourishment and passes waste materials.

urethra (yoo-REE-thruh). The duct through which urine passes out of the body from the bladder. In males, the urethra is also a part of the reproductive system, serving as a passageway for semen.

uterus (YOO-tuhr-uhs). The muscular, hollow, pear-shaped organ in females in which babies grow and are nourished before birth. Also called the womb.

vagina. A passage leading from the uterus to the outside of the body. Receives the erect penis during sexual intercourse, and allows a baby to pass from the womb and out of the mother's body during delivery. Also referred to as the birth canal. (box, cunt)

vas deferens (VAZ DEHF-uhr-uhnz). The tube in the male through which sperm passes from the epididymis to the seminal vesicles and urethra. Also called the spermatic or sperm duct.

vasectomy (vah-SEHK-tuh-me). The surgical procedure for sterilization in males. On both sides of the scrotum, a small incision is made and the sperm duct or vas deferens is cut, tied, sealed, or otherwise blocked off. Normal ejaculation of semen continues, but the semen no longer contains sperm. Sperm continue to be produced but they are reabsorbed by the body.

vulva (VUL-vuh). The external sex organ of the female. Includes the labia, clitoris, and the openings to the vagina and urethra. (beaver, pussy, snatch, slit, twat)